MANUAL OF CANCER TREATMENT RECOVERY

WHAT THE PRACTITIONER NEEDS TO KNOW AND DO

Stewart B. Fleishman, MD

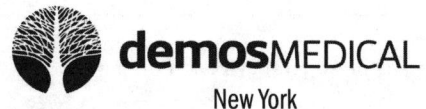

demosMEDICAL

New York

ISBN: 978-1-936287-31-4
e-book ISBN: 978-1-617050-61-9

Acquisitions Editor: Rich Winters
Compositor: Absolute Service, Inc.

Visit our website at www.demosmedpub.com

Medicine is an ever-changing science. Research and clinical experience are continually expanding our knowledge, in particular our understanding of proper treatment and drug therapy. The authors, editors, and publisher have made every effort to ensure that all information in this book is in accordance with the state of knowledge at the time of production of the book. Nevertheless, the authors, editors, and publisher are not responsible for errors or omissions or for any consequences from application of the information in this book and make no warranty, express or implied, with respect to the contents of the publication. Every reader should examine carefully the package inserts accompanying each drug and should carefully check whether the dosage schedules mentioned therein or the contraindications stated by the manufacturer differ from the statements made in this book. Such examination is particularly important with drugs that are either rarely used or have been newly released on the market.

Library of Congress Cataloging-in-Publication Data

Fleishman, Stewart.
Manual of cancer treatment recovery : what the practitioner needs to know and do / Stewart B. Fleishman.
    p. ; cm.
 Includes bibliographical references and index.
 ISBN 978-1-936287-31-4—ISBN 978-1-61705-061-9 (e-book)
 I. Title.
 [DNLM: 1. Neoplasms—psychology. 2. Neoplasms—rehabilitation. 3. Neoplasms—therapy. 4. Survivors. QZ 200]

   616.99′4—dc23

                2011044408

Made in the United States of America by Bang Printing.

11 12 13 14 15 5 4 3 2 1

Contents

PATIENT AND FAMILY WORKSHEETS

Foreword

From my vantage point as a head and neck surgeon whose practice is devoted to patients with cancer, I often marvel at the efforts that patients and their families make to get better. Rigorous radiation therapy and chemotherapy, often in combination with surgery of varying complexity have led to improved survival rates. Guiding each patient through the process of healing has likewise become more complex. Until now.

In the **Manual of Cancer Treatment Recovery: What the Practitioner Needs to Know and Do,** Dr. Fleishman has set forth a logical step-by-step system arising from growing literature of cancer survivorship. Written for the provider, whether in a solo community-based practice or at a large cancer research hospital, the *Manual* helps us to focus our efforts where they can make the most impact, and efficiently treat our patients. Whether considered as a stand-alone text or used in conjunction with the patient's book, **Learn to Live Through Cancer: What You Need to Know and Do,** this *Manual* provides a template for after-care that is more than an epilogue at treatments' end. It will influence the way you practice through preventive action, rather than reaction.

Every new or seasoned practitioner can dip into this rich resource to streamline the advice we give to patients as they become symptomatic, or more correctly, even before the symptoms become burdensome. Dr. Fleishman distills almost thirty years' experience into a plan that can easily be adapted to an individual patient. Using his training as a high school biology teacher, he has worked to both help us anticipate patients' needs, the questions patients are likely to ask, and their solutions.

Having sensitized us to the particular challenges of survivorship, the Institute of Medicine Report, *From Cancer Patient to Cancer Survivor: Lost in Transition* has likewise challenged us to tighter patient surveillance and clearer communication with each other. The forms and model discussions in this *Manual* make it easier for us to answer the IOM's call and integrate these practices into our practices. Many of us attended medical school before seminars in communication were included in the curriculum. Breaking good news, or bad, or informing a family that someone is critically ill is something we learned only by modeling our mentors. Though we prescribe opioids to better treat cancer pain, when have we thought through a plan to taper a patient comfortably? Do we have a similar plan to ease a patient off benzodiazepine antiemetics to avoid unnecessary emergency calls or visits? Do we have a step-wise approach to preventing or treating constipation or diarrhea during treatment? Is weight maintenance a parameter we track and for which we intervene aggressively? Now we do.

This book gives you the tools to incorporate logical and time-tested treatment plans for your use every day. It is like having Dr. Fleishman at your shoulder during rounds.

His vast training and experience, combined with his sensitivity towards patients' needs throughout this stressful period, provides us with a focus and direction that often falls short of our true potential to help. Using these tools in direct patient care and with trainees will improve patient care as well as your daily professional satisfaction in oncology.

Mark S. Persky, MD
Chairman, Department of Otolaryngology—Head and Neck Surgery, Beth Israel;
Interim Chairman, St. Luke's-Roosevelt;
Physician-In-Chief, Continuum Otolaryngology—Head and Neck Surgery Service Line
Professor of Clinical Otolaryngology, Albert Einstein College of Medicine, New York

Preface

The *Manual of Cancer Treatment Recovery: What the Practitioner Needs to Know and Do* presents the first comprehensive program to guide the recovery from cancer and its treatment. This innovative program focuses on the maintenance of quality of life at the time of diagnosis and runs in tandem with treatment, rather than beginning when treatment is completed. It "upstreams" symptom management to minimize cachexia, deconditioning, and much of the distress that accompanies having cancer.

This book, along with the patient and family-focused *Learn to Live Through Cancer: What You Need to Know and Do*, provides practical information to help patients, families, and the treatment team anticipate needs before they arise. The *Manual* provides easy-to-use forms that your patients may complete before the Initial Consultation, tools to improve communication between you and other providers and survivorship care plans to pass information to primary care providers after treatment is completed. Model discussions at transitional points in care are featured, useful to new practitioners and those who mentor fellows, house staff, advance practice nurses, and oncology social workers.

The *Manual* and *Learn to Live Through Cancer* feature a way for you, your staff and your patients to structure your collective efforts efficiently. These monographs introduce **The LEARN System,** promoting a five-point framework for patients to organize their endeavors:

Living: identifying something that makes life meaningful, enjoy oneself or help others during the week when not attending treatment;

Education: learning something new each week about one's cancer and recovery;

Activity: incorporating a practical at-home or supervised movement or exercise plan to minimize fatigue and deconditioning, taking co-morbidities into account;

Rest and Sleep: adapting techniques from sleep researchers to improve rest and sleep to maintain daytime energy; and

Nutrition: maintaining oneself as close as possible to ideal body weight, avoiding cachexia or hormone-related weight gain.

The *Manual* puts tools in your hand that respond to both the 2006 Institute of Medicine report *From Cancer Patient to Cancer Survivor: Lost in Transition* as well as the proposed changes to the standards of the *American College of Surgeons Commission on Cancer* which may feature the use of survivorship care plans and the routine assessment of palliative care and psychosocial needs.

Clinicians will appreciate the systematic approach to the treatment of symptoms that do not yet have widely accepted guidelines, such as tapering patients from opioid analgesics or benzodiazepine antiemetics, and the treatment of constipation and diarrhea.

It is hoped that use of this *Manual* will streamline the efforts you and your staff invest in guiding your patients through their journey through modern, multimodal, interdisciplinary cancer treatment.

Acknowledgments

An endeavor such as this guide is very definitely not a one-man show. Thousands of people—colleagues, patients, families, and good friends—have taught me what I am passing on here. I have been blessed with mentors in my personal and professional life who have given me access to a fount of information and taught me the skills to cobble the facts together, all while inviting me to be a part of their journey. Their altruism works in that they, too, can "give forward" through my efforts, benefiting countless others from their experience. Mentioning names means I may omit some meaningful ones, so please excuse any omission.

First, to my parents Mariane and Bill for rooting me in the technical aspects of our family pharmacy, fostering the abilities to communicate effectively and diplomatically, and prioritizing "helping others" as a core life value; my family: Bruce, Herbert, Iris, Jeffrey, Sharon, Severine, Lynne, Nan, David, Ira, Naomi, and Linda in this lifelong journey in which we have found that the more you give, the more you get.

Next, to my medical mentors—Doctors (all): Jimmie Holland, who is the founder of the field of psycho-oncology and mentor par excellence; Mary Jane Massie who taught me how to clarify the message; Lynna Lesko, Kanti Rai, Ronald Blum, Arthur Sawitsky, Louis Harrison, Mark Persky, Moses Nussbaum, Roy Sessions, Russell Portenoy, Manjeet Chadha, Suzan Naam, Kenneth Hu, Sheldon Feldman, Jean-Marc Cohen, Warren Enker, Martin Karpeh, Roy Sessions, Wendi Lovenvirth, Andrew Evans, Ronald Ennis, Stephen Malamud, Bruce Culliney, Peter Kozuch, Seth Cohen, Sharon Rosenbaum-Smith, Susan Boolbol, Laurie Kirstein, Mark Smith, Arnold Katzoff, and Howard Berkowitz who all put theory into practice every day to save and improve so many lives, then teach us all how to do what they do; and Sarah Schwartzbord Gelberd who has helped me to clarify, question, nurture, and learn over more than 30 years of camaraderie.

To so many nonphysician colleagues that have taught me so much and set the bar higher and higher: Elise Carper, Thelma Myers-Navarro, Cindy Turkeltaub, Diane Serra, Diane Blum, Carolyn Messner, Victoria Rosenwald, Bridget Bennett, Darren Arthur, Nancy Bourque, Lori Schwartz, Carolyn Cassin, Anne Moses, Marilyn Bookbinder, Jason Bishop, Susan Gold, Carol Farkas, Neva Solomon, Nayo Akowe, Enid Stecker, Rosie Hylton, Damien Francois, Sandy Lansinger, Myra Glajchen, Christine Jones, Carol Lowe, Cesar Espineda, George Handzo, Randye Retkin, Howard Gelberd, and Deborah Korzenik whose oncology social work, nursing, nutrition, legal, and leadership skills embody the finest professional principles each and every day; Victoria Schlegel, Wendy Serkin, Stephanie Spinner, Barbara Brownell, Sue Fredericks, with extraspecial gratitude to Elayne Feldstein—wordsmith and thoughtsmith educator whose need to understand pressed me to understand more and explain better; our wonderful string of Continuum students with special mention to Dimitri Yukvid and Erica Silen for their help on the Survivorship Project and Jus Chadha on the nutritional section; Ellen Clegg and Allen Levine who put "chemo-brain" into my brain and into the daily lexicon.

And to scores of patients, some long-term cancer survivors and some not, whose trust and search for life after cancer has served as my beacon. Special mention to Jeffrey Fleishman, Barbara Brownell, and Elayne Feldstein whose own survivorship underscores that cancer affects all of us without exemption and whose personal and professional advice has helped disseminate this work into the print and electronic worlds.

Special mention to the grateful patients and foundations who have helped throughout my career to promote projects and services in order to afford me the opportunity to learn from patients, families, and colleagues. These include the Millman family, the New York Community Trust, the Pechter–Machis family, the Michelle Klipstein-Cohen Foundation, the Schnurmacher Foundation, the Nagorski family, the Brody family, the Alvin Smith family, the Sandford Simon family, the Stein Family/Balm Foundation, the Brodoff family, the Karpas family, the Joel Finkelstein Family Foundation, the American Cancer Society, the Cancer and Leukemia Group B cooperative clinical trials group, the American College of Surgeons Commission on Cancer, and the Federation of Jewish Philanthropies. Cancer research cannot be pursued in current times without the support from the pharmaceutical industries that have been able to foster some of my research without bias: Abbott-Ross, Celgene, Merck, Solvay, and Sapphire Corporations.

All of us providers are also patients during our lives. I would like to thank those who have helped my parts to work well enough to set these words to paper: Ben Zane Cohen, MD; Jay Wisnicki, MD; Suzanne Bellante, OD; Peter Halper, MD; David Gorman, MD; Donald Kastenbaum, MD; Nate Schulman, MD; Ira Finegold, MD; and Bruce Haber, DDS.

With the advances in cancer medicine and biology, perhaps all oncology specialists will seize the lion's share of symptom management and support when the majority of patients will present with curable diseases.

Thank you all.

A Few Words About Language

More than just political correctness, the treatment of cancer involves many people, and their titles are continually evolving.

To be concise without sacrificing inclusiveness, certain group identifiers are short-hand for a variety of titles. Please be assured that no one is being left out of the village that it takes to care for someone with cancer.

"**Provider**" encompasses physician, nurse, social worker, psychologist, pharmacist, optometrist, nutritionist/dietician, technician, tumor registrar, physical therapist, occupational therapist, speech or stoma therapist, research assistant, information specialist, patient navigator, pastoral care chaplain, educator, or volunteer. Cancer is a condition treated by professionals coming from a multitude of disciplines working together in an interdisciplinary manner. Their services can exist because of administrators, administrative assistants, policy makers, legislators, donors, and visionaries who all make our complicated system function.

"**Family**" or "**caregivers**" includes our nuclear families, blood relatives, marital families, extended family, friends who are our family of choice, neighbors, acquaintances, fellow congregants, fellow travelers, and anyone who extends their hand and largesse to us when we are in need, over the span of a lifetime, occasionally, or even just once.

In the spirit of gender equality, most times **he**, **she**, **he or she**, **he and she**, or **(s)he** should be read as acceptable surrogates for each other, unless clearly gender-specific.

So please read "provider" and "family" and gender-related pronouns in this wider context.

The following passage is in *Learn to Live Through Cancer: What You Need to Know and Do:*

The Fine Print

The information provided in this book is of general interest. Since the situations involving cancer and its treatment can vary from individual to individual, your providers can help you individualize the care, using what is pertinent for you. Be sure to check if any of the interventions discussed apply to you or not, or need to be customized in some way.

Introduction

▓ HOW TO USE THIS BOOK AND WHY IT IS IMPORTANT TO YOU

Progress in Cancer Diagnosis and Treatment Reveals New Needs

We all have too much to read and not enough time. Like all of my colleagues, I have the piles of journals ready to read with the best intentions in mind. But for many of us, thorough journal reading gets postponed when prioritizing a variety of professional and personal responsibilities.

Then why should anyone have the time to read (no less write) a new contribution to the piles? Patients, families, and advocacy groups have brought a persuasive message forward highlighting the need for specialty level of care for the growing number of cancer survivors. A perfect storm has been fueled by consumer advocacy coincident with the development of practice guidelines for medical subspecialties. Today, there is a true need for clinical care, health services research, and strategic planning in response to the increase in the number of survivors and their extended survival time.

The Institute of Medicine Report, From Cancer Patient to Cancer Survivor: Lost in Transition

One of the most convincing statements of this developing need is contained in the 2006 Institute of Medicine (IOM) report, *From Cancer Patient to Cancer Survivor: Lost in Transition.* The IOM report makes a scholarly case for the oncology community to work together to improve the period of survivorship. Both the National Coalition for Cancer Survivorship and the National Cancer Institute's Office of Cancer Survivorship have defined *survivor* in the broadest sense: *An individual is considered a cancer survivor from the time of diagnosis, through the balance of his or her life. Family members, friends, and caregivers are also impacted by the survivorship experience and are therefore included in this definition.**

Patients And Providers Echo the Same Message

As a physician with board certification in *hospice and palliative medicine* and with fellowship training in *psycho-oncology*, my professional opportunities have taken me to the very beginning of the continuum of survivorship, working in academic cancer centers to define and provide care for patients in the midst of initial diagnostic testing, carrying through surgery, chemotherapy, and radiation therapy. Mentorship from the "giants" in these fields, with an early career chance to become an investigator in the Cancer and

Leukemia Group B, it became clear that symptom management is provided from the first phone call onward, not just at end of life. Such a revolutionary concept crystallized quite early and helped define my 25-year career path, research interests, and teaching agenda. As with many good things in life, being in the right place at the right time expedited the opportunities that were granted through training and practice. Combined with mentoring from role models with **boldface names**, this work is possible.

The need for good information in symptom control was repeated in many settings. When we had presented the results of a study of fatigue and cognitive impairment after chemotherapy at the San Antonio Breast Cancer Symposium, many colleagues asked where they could get information both for themselves and to distribute to patients. One medical oncologist from the Seattle-Tacoma area said, "Patients mention that these things happen, but I do not know what to tell them."

Cancer*Care*, the New York-based agency runs the very successful Cancer*Care* Connect Teleconferences on a variety of topics each month. They are telephone-based, call-in programs about an hour in length and free to both the public and professional caregivers. Calls attract between a few hundred participants and about 4,000. When I had the honor of presenting on the heavily attended teleconference about cancer cachexia, the same sentiment was echoed. The same request was repeated on other calls about cognitive impairment and fatigue during the *Questions and Answers* segment of the conference. Other participants' comments resonated, "My oncologist says she is not familiar with what you are talking about. Is there a book or reference I can give them?" and "No one knows what I am talking about out here."

New Solutions Needed to "Bend the Cost Curve of Cancer Care"

Smith and Hillner[†] have suggested changes in attitude and practice in their powerful *The New England Journal of Medicine* editorial, *Bending the Cost Curve in Cancer Care.* Two of the four suggested changes in providers' attitude and practice can be operationalized using *My Recovery Plan* and *The LEARN System.* Using one of the worksheets, *What Is Important to Me*, and the early introduction of a symptom management focus gives "doctors and patients more realistic expectations" and "better integrates palliative care into usual, concurrent care." These issues addressed by Smith and Hillner dovetail nicely with the approach set forth in this Manual. As thought leaders in oncology, their vision for the future involves high-quality interventions that are careful with health care dollars.

A Confluence of Opportunities

When the New York Community Trust funded Ronald Blum, MD, and our team at the Continuum Cancer Centers of New York (Beth Israel and St. Luke's-Roosevelt) to develop personal health record (PHR) for patients receiving multimodal treatment for head and neck cancer, we built in a provider's tutorial to anticipate and meet this need.

The sum of these experiences—and through thousands of patient and family encounters over the years—has underscored the need to incorporate healing and recovery from the very start of care. When I would address the steps to take to recover after often an extended period of chemotherapy and radiation therapy, patients and families often responded with a puzzled expression and often responded, "How come any of you didn't mention all of this earlier?" Such responses as these sparked discussion and pilot programs at cancer centers around the country. Design of sound clinical trials would be needed to identify the clinical issues and best practices to ameliorate them. The issue of early attention to symptom management was addressed at the 2004 National Institutes of Health–sponsored *State-of-the-Science Conference on Symptom Management in Cancer: Pain, Fatigue, and Depression*, concluding that attention to these symptoms be given attention over the trajectory of cancer illness.[‡]

What exactly are the liabilities in working on wellness right from the start of care? Would the bleeding risks of thrombocytopenia or the risk of pathologic fracture be significant enough to discourage graduated activity? Would maintaining the proper food intake minimize weight loss in cancer cachexia or the predictable weight gain often seen with hormonal treatments in breast and prostate cancers? As patients are increasingly treated in ambulatory settings and resting more at home during chemotherapy and radiation therapy, can we offer more effective guidance than a benzodiazepine prescription?

American College of Surgeons Commission on Cancer Ratifies New Guidelines Including Survivorship Programs and Routine Assessment of Palliative Care and Psychosocial Needs

The Commission on Cancer has updated their guidelines for 2012 and forward with standards that widen the scope of treatment provided in its accredited centers to embrace three of the areas that this book covers: survivorship, distress, and palliative care needs. With a phase-in of these "new" standards, systems that measure and track these important clinical services are now part of the comprehensive treatment we are to provide for an individual with cancer. The principles and strategies in this book can be adapted to these new guidelines.

Common Goals of General Health and Healthy Heart Guidelines

When looking at the literature, evidence can be found for a burgeoning interest on each of the components of healing separately, but not for a bundled package. We already advise patients about each of the parameters in a nonuniform manner and often as an afterthought. Colleagues in other specialties such as in cardiology have adopted preventive guidelines for the general public to minimize heart disease. Federal guidelines for good eating and physical activity exist for the general public. Not surprisingly, the advice for eating well and exercise for the general public and that to maintain heart health are similar to the suggestions we offer to cancer survivors.

Instead of trying to reinvent the proverbial wheel, what is needed is a system to present to patients in a variety of treatment settings that vary from a sliding scale clinic or county-based hospital to small community-based hospitals and cancer centers, or academic cancer research hospitals and prestigious private practices. Assembling a team of cancer-wise colleagues directly available in physical therapy, nutrition, social work, pastoral care, psychology, and patient education is a luxury, limited to larger centers and practices. Getting patients to appointments with each of these clinicians in a coordinated way is a challenge in any setting. Initiating referral authorizations through insurance carriers is further impediment to uniform referral. Patient availability through weekly chemotherapy or 5-day-a-week radiation therapy appointments is a real obstacle.

Those of us charged with treating cancer have yet to develop a fully effective approach. Often on the fly, printouts and directions are given to patients. Their importance often loses to the triage of neutropenia or anemia. Why not then has a method that involves patients and families from the start in their own recovery? *My Recovery Plan* fills that void, having patients think about, discuss, and even document their personal preferences of communication style and values that have taken root *before their cancer diagnosis* and will endure well afterward. Using a mnemonic, a guiding feature of *My Recovery Plan* is The LEARN System. Such a system not only meets and exceeds the standard to promote effective patient education.

Companion to a Patient-Centered Program

This *companion manual* is paired to the book written specifically for patients and families, *Learn to Live Through Cancer: What You Need to Know and Do*. It features *My Recovery Plan* and *The LEARN System*.

The LEARN System brings together the concept to intervene early on symptom management in a format that helps organize one's information and tasks as a *new* cancer survivor. It is designed with the most liberal definition of *survivor* in mind, beginning at the time of diagnosis and following through a period of disease-free survivorship or recurrence/relapse. *My Recovery Plan* featuring The LEARN System focuses on information that patients and families can and need to learn during treatment from their providers about their particular clinical course, with an emphasis on five basic tasks:

L – focus regularly on an aspect of **li**ving outside of the treatment with a broader life perspective

E – **e**ducation; learning as much as fits your style about one's cancer and its treatment to expedite recovery

A – physical **a**ctivity to the extent able during and after treatment minimizes deconditioning afterward

R – using periods of **r**est and energy conservation to optimize energy during and after treatment

N – good **n**utrition paired with the limitations of treatment to maintain lean body mass, energy, and healing

The LEARN System organizes what we often ask patients to do in a more formal way and provides some tools for patients and families to do so.

Components of The LEARN System

L	Living
E	Education
A	Activity
R	Rest
N	Nutrition

One goal of this manual is to review the growing evidence for weight maintenance, exercise, optimizing energy, and targeted education to ease one's time during treatment and promote recovery. With the disparate use of various versions of written and electronic medical records, it is often the patient and family who transmit real-time information between providers at follow-up visits that occur before reports can be written and transmitted. (The need for such communication tools were made clear during the Head & Neck Cancer PHR Project.)

My Recovery Plan encompasses The LEARN System's goals. Through a set of patient-and provider-friendly forms, enhances communication, weekly planning, and goal setting in a way that is not threatening or scary. Just as a personal financial plan does not start out with being destitute, a survivorship program does not start with end of life and work backward. Lots of planning and living occurs between a first paycheck and financial independence or bankruptcy. Similarly, lots of planning and living occurs between the day of a cancer diagnosis and disease-free survival or the end of life.

This manual will summarize the salient points for clinical practice found in the IOM report and suggest a system of care that is "value added" to the treatment patients currently receive in a variety of settings, from large tertiary care academic centers to community-based oncology practices and clinics that treated underserved, underinsured patients with cancer. It will familiarize providers with the theory and work sheets easily so that participation is collaborative.

Throughout the patient book, *Learn to Live Through Cancer: What You Need to Know and Do, My Recovery Plan* features tools for self-assessment and accountability and those that improve communication between patient and a myriad of providers. To ease provider familiarity with these forms, information on their use is featured in this manual. Ideally, using this manual and the patient-centered book together with your patients would coordinate the job. Working from this manual on its own can serve to funnel the information through you and your staff.

To meet the modern modes of communication which is no longer centered on paper communication but online, an associated Web site, http://www.cancer knowanddo.com, will bring electronic communication tools and up-to-the-minute information that may be newer than a published book. A provider's blog will give a forum for providers to share information about The LEARN System and updates.

▨ PRINCIPLED RECOVERY EFFORTS REACH
THE SAME CONSENSUS

Whether your patients and their families use *Learn to Live Through Cancer: What You Need to Know and Do* or not, the principles set forth of planning, communication, activity, and good nutrition can be emphasized in your practice. For patients in the midst of treatment, feeling like one has a purpose and be a contributing member of society during treatment has very little downside. Eating properly to maintain lean body mass, having restorative rest and sleep, and being informed and physically active within realistic limits can help set a focus on recovery from the very start of care. If you work in an environment where these modalities of care are readily available and accessible by patients and families, you are well ahead of the pack. If your practice setting cannot offer these enhanced services, then this system can help you, your staff, and your patients.

▨ ENDNOTES

* Hewitt M, Greenfield S, Stovall E, eds. *From Cancer Patient to Cancer Survivor: Lost in Transition*. Washington, DC: The National Academies Press; 2005:29.

† Smith TJ, Hillner BE. Bending the cost curve in cancer care. *N Engl J Med.* 2011;364(21):2060–2065.

‡ Kramer BS. The National Institutes of Health state-of-the-science conference on symptom management in cancer: pain, depression, and fatigue. *J Natl Cancer Inst.* 2004;32:1–158.

Section I

What You Need to Know
About Survivorship

Emerging Needs of Survivorship: Beyond The Institute of Medicine Report, *From Cancer Patient to Cancer Survivor: Lost in Transition*

In its landmark 2006 report, *From Cancer Patient to Cancer Survivor: Lost in Transition,* the Institute of Medicine (IOM)[1a] looks critically at the care needed for the steadily increasing number of cancer survivors. Because of the convergence of the advances in cancer treatment, health services research, and a heightened public health awareness, cancer has become a chronic illness with a growing prevalence. The increase in survival is owed in large part to the successful public health message of early detection and screening coupled with more effective treatment. In our current environment, this awareness welcomes health services research while the science of health care delivery enlightens us to the challenges of defining and coordinating optimal care after diagnosis and onwards. An increase in the number and longevity of survivors has brought us to look at the long-term outcomes of treatment and the care we provide to survivors and their families. Much of the information gathered is from an ever-growing vocal groundswell of survivors because toxicities of Grades I and II are underreported in follow-up from clinical trials. Their "anecdotal" reports have alerted investigators to clusters of subsyndromal consequences of cancer and its care that span physical sequelae and psychological adaptation affecting spiritual, vocational, and economic life after cancer. Falling "below the radar," only recently have these struggles been identified.

The report is a comprehensive description of the clinical needs of survivors and catalogues which services will be needed in the future along with the research agenda to refine the needs. The goal of the IOM report is to define and improve quality of care for survivors.

From Cancer Patient to Cancer Survivor identifies four of the "essential" components of survivorship care: prevention, surveillance, intervention, and coordination of care. It reports that cancer survivors are often lost to systematic follow-up within our health care system, and so, opportunities to effectively intervene are missed. Many people finish their primary treatment for cancer unaware of the information they—and their primary care providers—need to know, identifying the heightened health risks as a result of having cancer and treatment and planning for future health care needs. The IOM report focuses on what is needed now and what our fragmented delivery system can actually provide. The report underscores the lack of awareness of what, if anything, can be done to nurture recovery as well as minimize the late effects of cancer and/or treatment. It further characterizes that fragmentation in information among providers stifles effective communication and reduces provider awareness. Simultaneously, discussions of survivorship in the media and in existing educational materials will be increasing patients' and families' expectations.

Four Essential Components of Survivorship Care

The Institute of Medicine identified the following essential components of survivorship care in its report, *From Cancer Patient to Cancer Survivor: Lost in Transition*:

Prevention
Surveillance
Intervention
Coordination

The prescription written by the IOM panel involves the collaboration of clinicians, researchers, advocates, and policy makers to raise awareness and provide improved care after treatment. Specifically, the IOM report recommends that a *comprehensive care summary* be created and given to each patient at the end of treatment. It also suggests that better tools should be developed and tested to follow up with patients and optimally treat late effects.

Recommendations From the Institute of Medicine Report: *From Cancer Patient to Cancer Survivor: Lost in Transition*

Recommendation 1: Health care providers, patient advocates, and other stakeholders should work to raise awareness of the needs of cancer survivors, establish cancer survivorship as a distinct phase of cancer care, and act to ensure the delivery of appropriate survivorship care.

Recommendation 2: Patients completing primary treatment should be provided with a comprehensive care summary and follow-up plan that is clearly and effectively explained. This "Survivorship Care Plan" should be written by the principal provider(s) who coordinated oncology treatment. This service should be reimbursed by third-party payors of health care.

Recommendation 3: Health care providers should use systematically developed evidence-based clinical practice guidelines, assessment tools, and screening instruments to help identify and manage late effects of cancer and its treatment. Existing guidelines should be refined and new evidence-based guidelines should be developed through public and private sector efforts.

▨ WHAT CAN BE DONE *NOW*

The inherent delays in developing, field testing, and incorporating new tools of assessment or treatments into guidelines will delay their implementation for many years. The project also competes for an ever-shrinking pool of health care research dollars. In the interim, today's surviving patients will be left waiting for validation and reliability studies followed by clinicians' consensus. What is presented both here and in the patient-focused companion book *Learn to Live Through Cancer: What You Need to Know and Do* is an adaptation of tools and recommendations already in use, with an emphasis on patient and family involvement. The IOM report falls short in that it carefully examines the role of clinicians, researchers, and the health care delivery system but does not suggest which specific steps patients and families can take. The carefully considered and wonderful suggestions in the IOM report involve activities done for/to the patient. A number of suggestions that in 2005 were considered progressive have become routinized, even commonplace components of practice guidelines and everyday care. The responsibility is heavily weighted on providers. However, with the more active participation of patients and their caregivers in cancer treatment as in all other aspects of health, the responsibility of recovery and healing has become more collaborative. And patients feel more empowered.

The next logical step is to ask, **"What can a patient and family do *now*?"** What do patients and families need to know and do (or not do) to best rebound from cancer and restore their quality of life after cancer? Should we the providers suggest and guide? Otherwise, who should do so? What information do we have? How good is the information? Which tools have been already developed? What is the hazard of developing survivorship programs that may not have been fully vetted in clinical trials thus far? How can we all—providers, patients, and caregivers—adapt what we know about the recovery from other illnesses? What is the role of a formal survivorship plan that encourages active collaboration?

The gaps in the recommendations in *Lost in Transition* have been in large part the stimulus for the tools featured in this book. Whether a patient is treated in a private oncology office, clinic, community hospital, or large academic setting, access to specialized services is inconsistent.* Using *My Recovery Plan* and *The LEARN System* can bring such targeted services to patients and families under the provider's guidance.

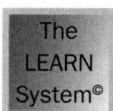

p. 143
My
Weekly
Recovery
Planner

Learn to Live Through Cancer: What You Need to Know and Do guides a patient and their family and caregivers through the initial process of diagnosis and treatment with a special focus on recovery. The tools contained reveal helpful information because it is useful from the very beginning with referral to cancer specialists for an initial consultation. The materials help the patient unfamiliar with the multidisciplinary nature of cancer treatment understand the initial steps taken. Forms and checklists help a patient prepare for each step.

---

*As a surveyor to accredit Cancer Programs of the American College of Surgeons Commission on Cancer, I have been privileged to view many of our country's best practices. This experience has also allowed me to identify areas to adapt to the growing needs of survivors.

With its emphasis on maintaining quality of life throughout the trajectory of treatment, *My Recovery Plan* guides patients in defining their personals goals for their care *early* in the process, something often and formerly relegated only to end-of-life care planning. Simple fill-in forms that can be used electronically or on paper help focus each patient on the elements of recovery from the beginning and throughout treatment. Straightforward forms are provided to help a patient navigate between cancer specialists who do not all access a unified electronic medical record. This information serves as a basis for the comprehensive *Personal Health Records*, which can be more easily completed by clinicians at the end of treatment, consistent with the IOM's recommendations. Each week, a patient (with caregivers) sets out a simple plan for himself or herself, built on the basic tasks of being a patient in cancer treatment and maximizing the quality of life when not directly attending to the needs of treatment. The LEARN System is an acronym for those elements: **L**iving, **E**ducation, **A**ctivity, **R**est, and **N**utrition.

The
LEARN
System©

p. 168
Your
Personal
Health
Record

The *Living* component asks patients each week to pinpoint something—at least one activity, person, task, or anything else—that gives their life meaning. When the side effects of treatment are endured, it helps to have a clear-cut reason to sustain oneself. Patients have found this simple technique supportive over time to maintain perspective on the short-term investments in quality of life that are made during treatment.

Education is used in the broadest sense, referring to the specific body of knowledge that each patient acquires from treatment staff, pamphlets, books, the Internet, and friends and neighbors. With only a minority of patients who seek any type of counseling during their cancer treatment, information that is usually traded in support groups, waiting rooms, or in counseling is part of the basic information that normalizes the experience of being treated. Because education is an ongoing process, the book stresses referring to reliable and up-to-date external sources to keep up with our fast-changing field.

Despite the usual stigma of using *exercise* as an important component of general health, *Activity* stresses the importance of movement to the extent that is possible and safe throughout the course of treatment to avoid the general deconditioning that is so prevalent as patients finish treatment. Activity has always been an informal part of care. How many times have we said to patients admitted to the hospital, "Be sure to take your IV pole and walk the length of the hallway today"? Activity has been shown to minimize the incidence of cancer as well as the prevalence of recurrence and has generally been regarded as safe and advisable, with many benefits as long as certain limitations are respected.

The importance of *Rest and sleep* to overall health during cancer treatment has been minimally studied. Extrapolation from general health and wellness principles applies to patients undergoing treatment. The myriad of reasons why rest and sleep are interrupted can easily be remediated early and throughout the course of treatment. With an eye to preventing or controlling cancer and its treatment along with age-related comorbidities, rest and sleep should be prominent in care planning throughout cancer treatment.

Routine and reliable *Nutrition* advice is difficult to provide in respect to the wide variation in patients' needs, the type of cancer, prediagnosis weight, and the type of treatment. Yet, with cancer-induced and cancer-associated weight loss (or weight gain) accounting for significant comorbidity, information, and guidance at the start of treatment is necessary. The LEARN System places great importance on eating both properly and well during treatment and afterwards.

Using the *Manual of Cancer Treatment Recovery: What the Practitioner Needs to Know and Do* and *Learn to Live Through Cancer: What You Need to Know and Do* will help cancer providers easily and conveniently offer carefully considered information and direction to patients and families, and will facilitate communication among providers not electronically connected through a unified electronic medical record. This *Manual* is designed to make it uncomplicated for providers to become familiar with the tools to adopt in their own practices.

2

Early Intervention to Improve Treatment Outcomes

WHEN SURVIVORSHIP BEGINS

It is expected that by 2020, there will be 18.1 million American cancer survivors.[1b] In 2004, the National Coalition for Cancer Survivorship helped define the concept of survivorship[2] as "the experience of living with, through, and beyond a diagnosis of cancer." Fitzhugh Mullan[3] through both personal experience and professional acumen described survivorship in "seasons":

1. **Acute survival** begins with the diagnosis of the illness and is dominated by diagnostic and therapeutic efforts. Fear and anxiety are important and constant elements of this phase.
2. **Extended survival** is a period during which a patient goes into remission or has terminated the basic, rigorous course of treatment and enters a phase of watchful waiting, with periodic examinations and "consolidation" or intermittent therapy. Psychologically, this time is dominated by fear of recurrence. This is usually a period of physical limitations because the tumor and treatment have exacted a corporal price. Diminished strength, fatigue, a reduced capacity for exercise, amputation of a body part, or hair loss may have occurred in the acute phase, but now they must be dealt with in the home, the community, and the workplace.
3. **Permanent survival** is roughly equated with "cure," but the person who has come through a cancer experience is indelibly affected by it. Problems with employment and insurance are common for persons who have been treated for cancer and are ready to resume a full life. The long-term, secondary effects of cancer treatment on health represent another area in which permanent survivors are at risk.

Defining the scope and needs of our future cancer populations is critical when thinking about health care delivery services and how to approach survivors' care. The Institute of Medicine (IOM) report, *From Cancer Patient to Cancer Survivor: Lost in Transition*, takes a very conservative approach to recommending when survivorship care should begin. The report proposes that an "organized plan for survivorship care should be developed by the time primary treatment ends." It defines *primary treatment* as the first course of therapy with the intention to cure cancer.[1a]

ADAPTATION OF EXISTING MODELS

Paralleling other advances in cancer medicine, it would be critical to test a model of early intervention. The interplay between the components—optimal nutrition, exercise, restorative sleep, and having good information—has not yet been studied in a patient population stratifying for type of cancer, stage, and treatment. As intellectually stimulating as such a study could be, it very well may be almost impossible to implement and quite impractical. Accrual and standardization between study sites to include a critical number of patients for the findings to be meaningful and then waiting the time for the data to mature to look at both short- and long-term effects would be a formidable task. The costs of such a study would be high in order to fund long-term follow-up, even though it would help validate a comprehensive model of care.

In this era of evidence-based medicine, much of our daily care is rooted in clinical experience rather than a placebo-controlled, randomized trial. The National Comprehensive Cancer Network (NCCN) struggled with this issue and established that even the most respected guidelines are largely developed with lower levels of evidence.[4]

An example of an attempt to look at one variable—exercise—was done by the Agency for Healthcare Research and Quality (AHRQ), formerly the Agency for Healthcare Policy and Research. The study reviewed a variety of behavioral interventions to modify physical activity in general populations, cancer patients, and survivors.[5] The report concluded that overall, the literature is positive, but the relative magnitude of the effect is difficult to judge given the wide range of outcomes examined. It called for more standardized measures and more studies examining longer outcomes. The 24 interventions reviewed indicate that physical activity is safe for cancer survivors and consistently results in improved physiologic and psychosocial outcomes.

The elements of The LEARN System that provide a hands-on, ready-to-go working model of care will be presented along with supporting evidence in the literature. It can be speculated that the power of the interactions between or among each of the components of The LEARN System can support each other if not magnify the benefits when used together.

How early should targeted recovery efforts begin?

Today's model needs to begin at the time of diagnosis, as asserted by Dr. Mullan. With hospital stays shortening and with the reality that some patients never experience a hospital admission over the course of their care, access to colleagues who can bring information to patients and families consistently and early becomes even more limited. Because many of the "supportive services," specifically patient navigators, specialized nutritional and social work counseling and physical/occupational therapists have limited reimbursement by third-party payors, preventive health maintenance during cancer treatment has not yet been mainstreamed. Patients and families consistently wonder why more complete information about diet and exercise were not supplied earlier in the course of care.

Theoretically, early adaptation of basic diet and exercise regimen tailored to the clinical limitations imposed by surgery, chemotherapy, and radiation therapy should improve both quality of life and reduce the morbidity of survivorship. Postoperatively, it is common practice to advance diet from *nothing by mouth (NPO)* to clear liquids, full liquids, and then solid foods as soon as a patient can tolerate it. After that, unless there are particular needs imposed by the cancer, such as instituting pancreatic enzymes or using a feeding tube, specific instructions are seldom supplied. Similarly, a patient will dangle his or her feet, sit in a chair, and walk the corridors as quickly as possible, with the next stage of instruction nonexistent or general such as "Do what you can."

There is no existing clinical trial examining which components are most beneficial, the optimal time such an intervention should begin, or which subset of patients stratified by age, gender, type of cancer, or treatment would benefit the most.

▨ UPSTREAMING PALLIATIVE CARE

Studies to look at better and earlier integration of symptom management and psychosocial support have looked to an existing model of palliative care. Despite our colleagues' misunderstanding that palliative care is synonymous with end-of-life care, it is a logical place to start from because the interventions of traditional palliative care *are the same as* those given earlier in treatment although they are called symptom management and psychosocial support.

Only recently has the timing of more traditional palliative care interventions (consult, pain management, goals of care discussion) been examined. Temel and colleagues[6] randomized 151 patients with newly diagnosed metastatic non-small cell lung cancer to an intervention that included teaching and discussion about illness and prognostic understanding, clarification of treatment goals, management of symptoms (pain, cough, dyspnea, fatigue and sleep disturbance, depression and anxiety, anorexia and weight loss, nausea and vomiting, constipation) with further appointments, and patient/family counseling. Quality of life, assessed using standard measures, improved. Median survival of the intervention group was significantly improved at 11.6 months versus 8.9 months ($P = .02$), even though the group received more aggressive care than the control group.

Bruera and Hui[7] make a compelling and eloquent case for an integrative model of palliative care and symptom management in assessment and treatment parallel to cancer. Schematics show how this model can be applied in a variety of practice settings, including a solo practice where the in-office resources are limited. The researchers compare having cancer with taking a car trip over a hazardous road with oil spills, accidents, and bumps in extreme heat. One can preserve a "hopeful and realistic attitude" in two scenarios: anticipating comfort and safety with air conditioning, seat belts, and airbags so that the journey can be safe and one can get to his destination. Preparation for having cancer likens palliative care techniques with safety and comfort measures that are common and mandatory.

THE SCOPE OF EFFORTS IN THE RECOVERY FROM CANCER

In *Cancer Rehabilitation: Principles and Practice*, Stubblefield and colleagues[8] have applied physiatric techniques to patients treated for cancer. In a comprehensive reference book, they cull the best practices for restoring function and quality of life to cancer survivors. The authors provide suggestions, identification, evaluation, and treatment of specific impairments and disabilities that result from both illness and treatment. In the groundbreaking textbook, *Handbook of Psychooncology: Psychological Care of the Patient with Cancer*[9] and subsequent revised editions, Jimmie Holland, MD, and many colleagues have catalogued the role of psychosocial interventions successfully applied to patients with cancer throughout the course of their care.

Reflecting the basic parts of The LEARN System, evidence exists for each element making a strong contribution to the recovery of quality of life after cancer, leaving aside the survival advantage that Temel's group found. The positive effects of diet and nutrition, exercise, and sleep have begun to undergo scrutiny to evaluate efficacy during and after cancer treatment. Patient and family education has been a hallmark in medical care for more than the last 30 years. Being mindful of one's actions and purposes (the "L" or Living component) and having a sense of the present and the future is a basic part of both Eastern and Western philosophies and not unique to cancer. The contributions of each when practiced together are yet to withstand clinical trial.

THE MODEL OF SYMPTOM CLUSTERS

The construct that looks at symptoms that occur simultaneously, or *symptom clusters* has garnered attention over the last few years. It is driven by the idea that each of the common symptoms associated with cancer and its treatment does not occur in isolation, but selected symptoms are often grouped with other symptoms. Separating which symptoms occur together clinically from those symptoms that relate to each other statistically on questionnaire-based assessments remains puzzling, although certain symptoms, such as "nausea–vomiting," "anxiety–depression," and "cough–dyspnea" are evident on both clinical observation and in research investigation. "Fatigue–pain" and "fatigue–insomnia–pain" have also been demonstrated statistically as clusters. Another proposed cluster is "depression–fatigue–pain."[10] Cheung and colleagues established a relationship among fatigue, poor general well-being, and decreased appetite; fatigue, drowsiness, nausea, decreased appetite, and dyspnea; and anxiety–depression.[11] In 2002, the National Institutes of Health convened a *State-of-the-Science Conference on Symptom Management in Cancer* and selected pain, depression, and fatigue as the symptom cluster most worthy of examination in its report published as a monograph for the National Cancer Institute.[12] The panel concluded that there was insufficient evidence to support the concept of symptom clusters. More significantly, they concluded that too many cancer patients receive inadequate assessment and treatment for pain, depression, and fatigue, and that clinicians should be more proactive in assessing their patients *throughout the course of illness.*[*] These findings remain current today and are part of the impetus for this book and The LEARN System.

Clinically, dyads, triads, or multiple combinations more predictably appear with certain cancers and at certain points during or after treatment in varying degrees. These patterns change as newer systemic or local therapies are developed.

ASSESSMENT OF SYMPTOMS USING STANDARDIZED TOOLS EASE OFFICE PRACTICES

Whether you practice in a single-practitioner office based in the community—a multispecialty practice, a community hospital, university-based hospital, or sliding scale clinic—one universal constant abides in all settings. Most patient encounters, when eye meets eye, almost always start with, "How are you?" Such an innocent inquiry can have distinct meaning for our patients. Some realize it is a socially correct opening line and say, "Fine" or "Okay." Others, whose emotions are more raw, say, "How do you expect me to feel? I have cancer!" with an exasperated tone. More assertive patients, in concert with assertive family members or friends who accompany them will say "(S)he is feeling terribly," or even pantomime behind the patient to speak with you, privately, outside of the room to relay their observations.

When the NCCN began to develop practice guidelines in the 1980s, a multidisciplinary panel was charged with translating the "How are you?" experience into something measurable that could be replicated across sites in parallel to treatment pathways. Out of these efforts[**] came the Distress Thermometer.

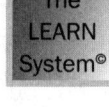

The Distress Thermometer can be used at *pivotal visits*. It is ideally given to patients on their way into their appointments, perhaps in the waiting room where they have a few minutes to think about their response. Attaching the information to the day's medical record entry either on paper or electronically can be an enormous help in a busy practice. If your office uses paper-based records, often the whole chart or day's progress notes and lab results are placed facedown to protect privacy near the entry way or on a chart holder in the door itself. The Distress Thermometer can be the day's cover sheet, and with a quick glance over the single page before entry to the room, you and your staff can get a global sense of how the patient is feeling and if the visit will be routine or challenging.

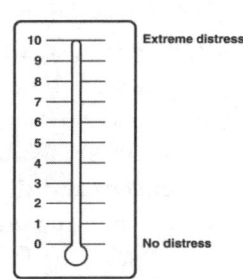

p. 142
Distress
Thermometer

---

[*]In the spirit of full disclosure, I was both on the planning committee and a presented *Treatment of Symptom Clusters: Pain, Depression, and Fatigue.*

[**]To continue in the same spirit of full disclosure, I have been and currently am a member of the NCCN Distress Management Panel, participated in the original validity and reliability study, and have used the Distress Thermometer in practice since 1999.

Although there is one global score, all items do not have the same importance. The global score does, though, flag the level of distress for fuller triage. No different than a 0–10 pain score, the global score is designed to fall into one of three categories for ease and quick triage:

0–3 Routine care, information given

4–6 Needs attention within a short period; a staff member can help with information or referral after the visit or call back in the following days

7–10 More completely assess during the visit; referral to multidisciplinary specialists

It is vital to note that the Distress Thermometer or a similar tool is a *triage tool* to help easily summarize a patient's immediate concerns.

When the concept and tool were first introduced, there was great concern among colleagues that asking about such personal information would "open Pandora's box" and actually lengthen the office visit or expose matters that could not be handled in an office practice. These concerns have not at all been realized in many years' use of the Distress Thermometer. Depending on your practice setting, other staff—particularly nurses, social workers, or inclined office managers—are the most knowledgeable about community-based resources and are eager to help. Their job satisfaction can actually improve if they see themselves as contributing to the greater good of the patient and family. As with other innovations in medical practice, adopting the tool is a slow process.

AHA* 2006 Diet and Lifestyle Recommendations for Cardiovascular Disease Risk Reduction[13]

- Balance calorie intake and physical activity to achieve or maintain a healthy body weight.
- Consume a diet rich in vegetables and fruits.
- Choose whole-grain, high-fiber foods.
- Consume fish, especially oily fish, at least twice a week.
- Limit your intake of saturated fat to <7% of energy, *trans* fat to <1% of energy, and cholesterol to <300 mg/day by
  - choosing lean meats and vegetable alternatives;
  - selecting fat-free (skim), 1% fat, and low-fat dairy products; and
  - minimizing intake of partially hydrogenated fats.
- Minimize your intake of beverages and foods with added sugars.
- Choose and prepare foods with little or no salt.
- If you consume alcohol, do so in moderation.
- When you eat food that is prepared outside of the home, follow the AHA Diet and Lifestyle Recommendations.

---

*AHA, American Heart Association.

> **Eat a Healthy Diet, With an Emphasis on Plant Sources Nutrition and Physical Activity Guidelines for Cancer Prevention: Summary of American Cancer Society Recommendations for Individual Choices**
>
> **Choose foods and beverages in amounts that help achieve and maintain a healthy weight.**
>
> - Pay attention to standard serving sizes (see "What counts as a serving?" table under the section, "Maintain a healthy weight throughout life"), and read food labels to become more aware of the number of actual servings you eat.
> - Eat smaller portions of high-calorie foods. Be aware that "low fat" or "non-fat" does not mean "low calorie," and that low-fat cakes, low-fat cookies, and other low-fat foods are often high in calories.
> - Switch to vegetables, fruits, and other low-calorie foods and beverages to replace calorie-dense foods and beverages such as French fries, cheeseburgers, pizza, ice cream, doughnuts and other sweets, and regular sodas.
> - When you eat away from home, choose foods low in calories, fat, and sugar, and avoid large portion sizes.
>
> **Eat five or more servings of vegetables and fruits each day.**
>
> - Include vegetables and fruits at every meal and for snacks.
> - Eat a variety of vegetables and fruits each day.
> - Limit French fries, snack chips, and other fried vegetable products.
> - Choose 100% juice if you drink vegetable or fruit juices.
>
> **Choose whole grains over processed (refined) grains and sugars.**
>
> - Choose whole grain rice, bread, pasta, and cereals.
> - Limit intake of refined carbohydrates (starches) such as pastries, sweetened cereals, and other high-sugar foods.
>
> **Limit intake of processed meats and red meats.**
>
> - Choose fish, poultry, or beans instead of beef, pork, and lamb.
> - When you eat meat, choose lean cuts and eat smaller portions.
> - Prepare meat by baking, broiling, or poaching rather than by frying or charbroiling.

There are a host of other standardized scales that assess symptom burden and quality of life when living with cancer. More suited for clinical research, they are not triage tools but stand-alone questionnaires tested for reliability and validity.

▪ COMMON GROUND WITH CARDIOVASCULAR DISEASE RISK REDUCTION RECOMMENDATIONS

Because cancer treatment occurs as a piece of our total health care, matching the goals of general health and cardiac health with cancer is more important than ever. The increase in the number of cancer survivors and length of the survivorship period affords an opportunity to better coordinate specialists' and generalists' recommendations. Not at all a surprise, the nutritional recommendations for the general population, the cancer population, and the prevention of heart disease are so similar, they're almost identical. Cancer-specific recommendations are described in Chapter 12 and detailed in the Appendix.

▓ COMMON GROUND WITH DIETARY GUIDELINES FOR AMERICANS 2010

Similar nutritional guidelines have been produced in a joint project between the US Departments of Agriculture and Health and Human Services that share the philosophy and details of the American Heart Association (AHA) and American Cancer Society (ACS) guidelines:

Dietary Guidelines for Americans, 2010[14]

- Prevent and/or reduce overweight and obesity through improved eating and physical activity behaviors.
- Control total calorie intake to manage body weight. For people who are overweight or obese, this will mean consuming fewer calories from foods and beverages.
- Increase physical activity and reduce time spent in sedentary behaviors.
- Maintain appropriate calorie balance during each stage of life—childhood, adolescence, adulthood, pregnancy and breast-feeding, and older age.
- Reduce daily sodium intake to less than 2,300 mg and further reduce intake to 1,500 mg among persons who are 51 years and older and those of any age who are African American or have hypertension, diabetes, or chronic kidney disease. The 1,500 mg recommendation applies to about half of the US population, including children, and most adults.
- Consume less than 10% of calories from saturated fatty acids by replacing them with monounsaturated and polyunsaturated fatty acids.
- Consume less than 300 mg/day of dietary cholesterol.
- Keep trans-fatty acid consumption as low as possible by limiting foods that contain synthetic sources of trans fats such as partially hydrogenated oils and by limiting other solid fats.
- Reduce the intake of calories from solid fats and added sugars.
- Limit the consumption of foods that contain refined grains, especially refined grain foods that contain solid fats, added sugars, and sodium.

continued

---

continued

- If alcohol is consumed, it should be consumed in moderation—up to one drink per day for women and two drinks per day for men—and only by adults of legal drinking age.
- Increase vegetable and fruit intake.
- Eat a variety of vegetables, especially dark-green and red and orange vegetables and beans and peas.
- Consume at least half of all grains as whole grains. Increase whole-grain intake by replacing refined grains with whole grains.
- Increase intake of fat-free or low-fat milk and milk products such as milk, yogurt, cheese, or fortified soy beverages.[14]
- Choose a variety of protein foods, which include seafood, lean meat and poultry, eggs, beans and peas, soy products, and unsalted nuts and seeds.
- Increase the amount and variety of seafood consumed by choosing seafood in place of some meat and poultry.
- Replace protein foods that are higher in solid fats with choices that are lower in solid fats and calories and/or are sources of oils.
- Use oils to replace solid fats where possible.
- Choose foods that provide more potassium, dietary fiber, calcium, and vitamin D, which are nutrients of concern in American diets. These foods include vegetables, fruits, whole grains, and milk and milk products.

▨ ADVOCATE A *COMMON SENSE* APPROACH

The main thrust of these various sets of guidelines is the same. They are not specifically designed for use in cancer survivors, but with some practical adjustments, are fully applicable. Patients and families routinely ask about diet and exercise, and the advice given is intuitively adjusted to an estimate of fatigue, pain, possibility of skeletal related events (pathologic fractures), blood pressure, and history of arrhythmia. Use the same good common sense and clinical judgment that applies when suggesting a more targeted approach in The LEARN System. Monitoring of a patient's general health status is routine throughout chemotherapy or radiation therapy without a departure from usual current practice.

▨ AN IMPROVED PARADIGM OF CARE

An improved paradigm of care involves instituting the clinical practices that will maximize healing *from the start of treatment.*

This graphic represents a more up-to-date model to be considered for newly diagnosed patients with cancer. With most cancer treatment provided in the ambulatory setting, the obstacles in the coordination of care is an opportunity to provide active attention to symptom management and supportive care throughout the trajectory of treatment as a distinct and important objective at all stages of care.

Section III contains more detailed information about using The LEARN System in your practice.

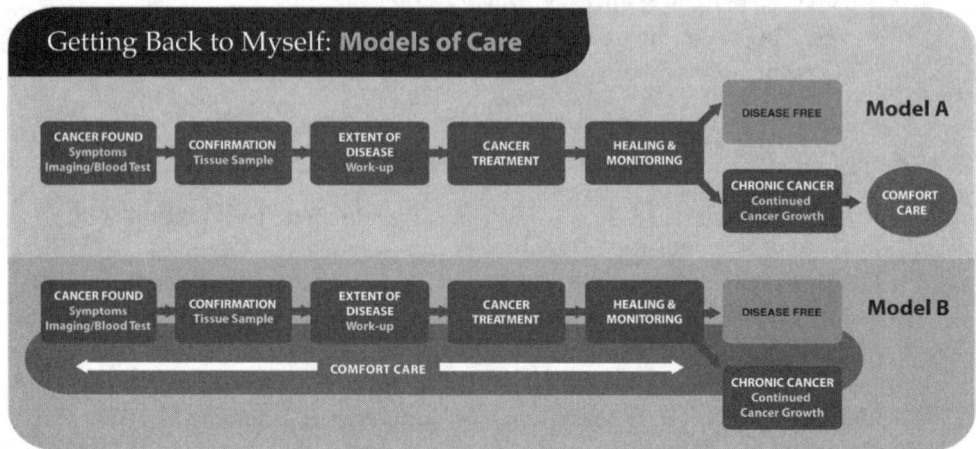

Model A: Comfort care recommended after chronic cancer is diagnosed. **Model B:** Comfort care included as part of treatment from initial diagnosis.

Section II

Implementing Effective Survivorship
Care in Practice

3

Apply Survivorship Tools *Early* in Care

The very mention of the concept of *goals of care* will probably evoke in many clinicians an association to end-of-life care. The term has been used euphemistically for discussions during which the idea of good response to treatment becomes remote, so the thoughtful clinician tries to help focus a patient and family on comfort that *can* be provided when extended survival becomes more and more dubious.

This unfortunate misassociation can delay an important discussion and prevent it from happening at the beginning of care. Mentioning goals of care may even bring a family to the erroneous implication that the situation is far more hopeless than it is. The term needs to be more widely applied throughout the course of cancer. Although one's goals may change with advancing illness and fear, basic enduring values are often timeless.

Some providers do get a sense of how patients make decisions early on through the use of *shared decision making*. A provider who affirms the concept of shared decision making will leave a few minutes during the initial consultation to assess the extent that a patient and family want to be participatory in the decision making regarding care. The very introduction of an inquiry into the patient and family level of comfort with shared decision making confirms that a provider will engage in discussion, or else the questions would not be asked at all.

What Is Important to Me was developed as an easy stepping-off point that minimizes the in-office time necessary to start a good dialogue at the very beginning of care. It stresses values, as well as goals. A common barrier to initiating discussions about values is the concern that they will take a lot of time. The form, completed outside of your office and then discussed, has been developed to assess the amount of decision-making input a patient or family wants and to get a snapshot of how they live their lives. The content has been adapted from another tool, *Five Wishes*, to apply to the very start of care. *What Is Important to Me* asks a patient to think about his or her values and enduring goals before beginning to feel the effects of treatment. Patients and families can—and should—dialogue between themselves before or soon after the initial consult and discuss their basic expectations. The decision-making process borrows in part from the principles of financial planning. It asks someone to think about how much investment of immediate quality of life he or she is willing to sacrifice for an unclear outcome. Within that framework, patients get to think about the coming days and weeks or months as well as long-term survival, and if they believe they are willing to commit to maintaining themselves on a maintenance regimen if indicated.

Another often-debated point is included as a choice on the form: whether or not an invasive procedure or high tech care, such as ventilatory support, would be acceptable if it is for a reversible process. All of us know the common in-patient scenario when

The LEARN System©

p. 133
What Is Important to Me

The LEARN System©

p. 205
Five Wishes

a patient with nonpulmonary metastatic disease develops pneumonia and needs a respirator for a finite period of time. If the patient had completed an advance directive using broad parameters such as "no tubes," ventilation would be precluded unless it was clearly specified.

Supporting information such as general life outlook (optimism vs. pessimism) and individual strengths will help round out a snapshot of your patients that will be helpful to you as you get to know them and their family while making better use of limited office time.

With the many tasks of an initial consultation, it is unrealistic to attempt to discuss the points of *What Is Important to Me* all at once. The form is much more useful as a pre-discussion guide for patients and families, so that the summary of such a long and difficult discussion can be provided during the initial visit. The form does not replace good discussion with a provider. But it does serve as a "dashboard" that clarifies the information.

Apart from the standard legal principle that patients who sign advance directives may change their minds (and subsequent paperwork), patients and families need to be reminded that through discussion they may "change their mind," and may actually make a decision that is *not in accordance with their initial preferences.*

As with any advance directive for end-of-life care, the details spelled out in the form serve as good "evidence" of patients' preferences for care if they lose capacity to make their wishes known. Local state laws may vary on the status of an oral discussion at a later date overturning the previously written document.

In keeping with the theme of early intervention to strengthen quality of life, such discussions should happen earlier in the course of care than traditional. To avoid dwelling on the decisions once treatment preferences are expressed, patients may find it best to figuratively and literally file the documents away and get on with the process of living through the treatment in preparation for extended survivorship.

Consistent with most providers' experience with advance discussions, one system does not suit everyone. *What Is Important to Me* allows for more flexibility than the usual later discussion.

How can I learn to handle such discussions with care so many times each day?

Evidenced by what we have learned in medical or nursing school and forward, skills can be taught *and learned.* With the rise in consumerism in health care and an ever-growing reliance on technology, our patients and the public in general have asked us to intensify our focus on the human aspects of care, beginning with effective communication. Linguists have been studying the provider–patient interaction for almost 30 years, suggesting ways in which we can communicate more effectively. Thoughtful listening is an integral component of good communication.

Think about your first day in Physical Diagnosis as a third year medical student or in nursing school. The experience might have been earlier in training if you attended a school with a progressive curriculum, strong social mission, or both. All of us probably felt intimidated to learn such a complex task and do it well. Many of us began by doing what had gotten us that far already, using lists and memorization for focus and direction. This worked well, to a point. Being afraid to forget something, we focused on asking all the right questions, perhaps focusing more on the questions rather than the answers. We've all been there. Through the "retrospectoscope," we might see ourselves as training to do cross-examination in a legal hearing, firing off one good question after another to get a complete history. By midcareer, we can assume that bad habits have been broken and good ones nurtured. We should be at a point where we are speaking, hearing, and listening to our patients' responses so that we can put together a differential diagnosis and treatment plan simultaneous to reacting to the responses with empathy. This is a very tall order. The key concept is that we *hear and listen*, having the information we just processed drive the next question. What a different experience than that first day in Physical Diagnosis.

When rushed, the part of the process that gets shorted is the listening and response. Listening is the teachable skill integral to serious discussions. Responding then becomes a logical and individualized progression. Using these skills will help tremendously here.

Knowing that our original history and physical experience was list-based, two physician colleagues have developed a system in which one of the steps supports listening, like *an* enzyme in a chemical reaction. Walter Baile and Robert Buckman together accepted the challenges highlighted by an informal survey done by the American Society of Clinical Oncology in 1998. With funding from the National Cancer Institute for a study about overcoming the barriers to effective communication when breaking bad news to patients, they developed a system for fellowship training called *Oncospeak* which featured a pithy acronym, SPIKES.[15,16] With the professional maturation of a few generations of fellows and well-accepted publication in the *Journal of Clinical Oncology*, many of us beyond fellowship received SPIKES training at live meetings or on American Society of Clinical Oncology (ASCO) videoconferences. Dr. Buckman's celebrity status as a contributing writer to the satirical comedy group *Monty Python* added a certain caché that helped the program gain notoriety and acceptance.

What is important to communication is in its application. SPIKES techniques should not be limited to "breaking bad news," but can be applied in truncated form to virtually any medical visit with patients and families. The SPIKES mnemonic keys us in to what we should be doing so as not to "reinvent the wheel" with each encounter.

SPIKES: Breaking Bad News System of Communication in Cancer

SET up interaction

PERCEPTION of patient/family ("Tell me what you know so far")

INVITE RESPONSE to give information and discuss

KNOWLEDGE imparted

EXPLORE reactions, meaning for future, emotions

STRATEGIZE and SUMMARIZE

In the SPIKES system, we remember to *set up the interaction*. Making sure to be at eye level with patients and/or families is a hard thing to do if a patient is in bed. It often means sitting down, which also removes the perception of rushing because we can't leave a room in midsentence when we're sitting.

Start with some limited social conversation, and confirm it is a "good time" to continue. Then just as we were taught in history taking, start with what is known. So checking out *perception* cues us to summarize what is known to that point—"Tell me what you know so far" or "Let me summarize what we know so far. When you had trouble breathing, some tests showed. . . ."

Next, *invite a response* and advance the discussion with new findings and clinical developments through *knowledge* in the form of crisp explanation tailored to a patient's or family's education and openness.

The next part, *exploring* a patient's and family's reactions is where the hearing and listening come into good use. Slow down and try to understand their response and the emotion that is packaged with it. At this time, make a genuine not canned empathic response—"This may be hard for you to think about," or "I bet this is different news than we had hoped for"—come to mind when discussing end-of-life care. It may mean your reassurance that a rapid progression of disease is *not imminent*, and that you really want to understand how the current decisions at hand for treatment fit in with other life decisions. Think of the people who would rather have the sure thing more secured versus those who are more comfortable with a long shot. Use the restrictive laws in your state as a reason to learn preferences early, even though an emergency is not expected. Don't say what you don't believe.

The final part is a *summary of the strategy* in which the next steps are discussed consistent with the amount of shared decision-making consensus. That can mean anything from, "You're in charge, doc" to "My daughter works in pharmaceutical research, and I will ask her to read the literature first," with all shades of in-between.

Using SPIKES is a stepping-stone to learn your own style. You will develop your own variation.

So just as we got more experienced taking a history and in doing a physical that became more targeted with the information we need to know, SPIKES helps us break out the *how* from the *what*. We know the *what*. The *how* can be easily learned.

Outcome Is a "Win-Win"

The outcomes of effort to strengthen familiarity with a patient's goals of care using the tools suggested benefits everyone. Practice will be more satisfying with better communication. At the end of the day, you are likely to have a greater sense of accomplishment. The tools suggested will also ease your communication with other providers.

■ HOW TO APPLY *WHAT IS IMPORTANT TO ME* AND *SPIKES EARLY* IN CARE

It is virtually impossible to "script" in advance a quality discussion between a patient/family and provider. There are many variables. Here is one example of how the system works. The words you will use will be more yours than anyone else's.

Mrs. AJ, an 84-year-old woman is referred for an initial consultation by a breast surgery colleague to see if chemotherapy is warranted. She has had a fine needle aspiration and then a lumpectomy and sentinel node biopsy. Her markers show ER+ PR+ HER2/neu underexpressed. Sentinel nodes show micrometastases. She is somewhat frail, although the only significant comorbidities are hypertension and hypothyroidism, which are optimally controlled. She is here with her daughter and son-in-law. One son died from lung cancer 5 years ago. She was widowed 30 years before when her husband had a sudden cardiac death. What complicates the decision making is the biopsy report, which found small nests of perineural invasion. She will see your radiation colleague this afternoon.

Other medical history is noncontributory. Nonsmoker; drinks wine 1 to 3 small glasses a week. Medicines: levothyroxine, alendronate (Fosamax) weekly taken 30 minutes after omeprazole (Aciphex®), acetylsalicylic acid (ASA) 81 mg qd, calcium, vitamin D. Your exam reveals her lumpectomy scar healing well, moderate osteoporosis, and a midline abdominal scar from a cesarean delivery 60 years prior.

After the examination, Mrs. AJ joins her family in your consult room. She has some biases for chemotherapy because in her words, "she's a healthy old lady." Her daughter wants very much for her mother not to suffer as her brother did—especially when he died anyway.

Armed with *What Is Important to Me*, you scan over the document and see that she is an optimistic type who values her survival even more than her comfort. She also is willing to "invest" her immediate quality of life to live longer, and she likes to be involved in decision making. You begin.

<u>Provider:</u> I see from the documents you prepared that you want to be part of the decision-making process and would invest some up front comfort to extend your life. If we look at the predictive models, we see that an initial round of chemotherapy with two types of drugs, adriamycin and cyclophosphamide, would add a few percentage points of survival advantage. That means four cycles of chemotherapy given 3 to 4 weeks apart. It is the kind that will make you tired, and you will lose some hair, but you should be able to carry out most of your usual activities. You will be tired, have to drink extra fluids, and get blood tests so we can judge how to personalize the dose for you.

<u>Daughter:</u> My mother is clearly in charge here, and I would say she's a bright woman (laughing). Ma, is it worth going through chemotherapy to you with such a slim benefit? What are the alternatives?

Provider: Later in life, women often opt for hormonal treatments to suppress the small amount of estrogen that is still present in menopause. Apart from hot flashes that can get worse, there are minor effects to know about, including moodiness and a slight increase in uterine cancer many years later. Tamoxifen has been the standard, and it may also substitute for your bone strengthening medicine for a while. There are newer medications that are slightly easier on the side effects, though they would not substitute for the osteoporosis drug.

Daughter: What about the radiation therapy appointment later?

Provider: The radiation oncologist will probably offer extra radiation to the lymph nodes, but I wouldn't want to second-guess her. You should discuss it with her directly today. The surgeon may also suggest an additional surgery to take out a few more lymph nodes. Both of those can risk arm swelling but that's only in a minority of patients.

Patient: How quickly do I need to let you know? Is this something that is urgent?

Provider: You have a chance to think about all of this. After you see the radiation oncologist today, your situation will be discussed at a meeting where we are all present and review cases that involve hard decisions. That won't be until next week.

Daughter: Your reputation is outstanding, and you seem to understand our concerns. But we certainly would want a second opinion. I hope that's not offensive to you.

Patient: Oh, . . .

Provider: (*rifles through file to get to demographics*) That's standard operating procedure here. You'll get the benefit of the input from all of us after the tumor board meeting. So, let me see who your insurance carrier is, so we can make some suggestions for another opinion.

Idealized interchange, yes, but illustrative all the same. Having thought about the personal circumstances, level of involvement in decision making, and how much of in the way of side effects she would want to bear for a certain survival advantage, the patient in this scenario gave the provider more time to assess and assure, at a time when communication could be stilted because of fear.

Having the discussion based on the details in *What Is Important to Me* also eases the discussion about advance directives.

Provider: Seeing how prepared you are, Mrs. AJ, can I assume that you and your daughter have discussed who would make decisions for you if you become unable to talk for yourself? Not that I expect any serious complications from either treatment, but. . . .

Patient: Getting to my age makes me value good planning. Yes, we have discussed my daughter being my agent, and she knows what I would want about tubes and machines.

Provider: Any other questions? Let's get you the names for some medical oncologists for a second opinion. Will you call us afterwards so we can proceed?

Hesitation to Be Proactive

Some of us may have even trained to be less proactive, with the idea that it may encourage doubt or overwhelm a patient who has just found out about the cancer and is scared. Some colleagues even fear angry calls from other children not living close by, wanting to protect their parent (and themselves) by not mentioning anything negative, especially advance directives. The perception of litigation risk may add to the hesitation. A little discomfort at first avoids the really awkward phone calls toward end of life often times on the telephone in the middle of the night or in the midst of a crisis. An increased level of candor makes it easier all of the way through, although it seems like a lot of work up front at the time of the initial consultation.

The previous example is actually an easy one. It would be hard to feel as if there is little hope to offer to a patient and family when planning adjuvant treatment for a healthy although older woman. Much of the angst about decision making with progressive disease is unnecessary once these tools are used throughout care.

4

Comorbidities and Cancer Survivorship

▩ SPECIAL TOPICS IN MANAGEMENT DURING SURVIVORSHIP: SYMPTOMS AND COMORBIDITIES

As the period of survivorship lengthens, the treatment of symptoms and comorbidities has needed to adapt as well. The challenge arises in the treatment of pain, dyspnea, insomnia, and chronic low-level nausea. Because the mainstays in treatment of these conditions are end-of-life medications that can cause dependence or tolerance, prescribing them further "upstream" has patients taking them for longer time. Knowing how to safely and comfortably taper patients off opioids and benzodiazepines can be carefully accomplished. Attention to patients who have developed dependence on nicotine and alcoholic beverages likewise need to be eased into a sustained abstinence.

Pain

Pain management in cancer treatment today has been better standardized. General guidelines are often, but not always, followed. Developed over the past 20 years, the most concise and scholarly summary of cancer pain management is found in the National Comprehensive Cancer Network (NCCN) Adult Cancer Pain Guidelines.[17] The following basic principles are emphasized:

- Routine, regular, and comprehensive pain assessment
- A logical pharmacologic approach that begins with short-acting opioids and then converted where indicated into long-term preparations
- The use of adjuvant medications, nonpharmacologic treatments, interventional procedures, aggressive treatment of side effects, psychosocial support, and educational efforts and materials

Adherence to the guidelines or their principles remains spotty even though acceptance is growing, although common barriers persist in various treatment settings. These barriers include fear of addiction; difficulties in screening for past opioid dependence among patients who have not been honest about their history and then use opioids aberrantly; investigation by federal and state authorities into providers' prescribing practices; and the extra burden to monitor the use of opioids. A groundswell of advocacy is now underway to sanction providers who do *not* adequately treat pain.

Advocacy on behalf of patients by both providers and family members remains a consistent need. Knowing other providers with specific experience in cancer pain in your community is vital. Providers who have specialist-level facility with pharmacologic treatment, nonpharmacologic modalities (such as massage or biofeedback), and interventional procedures are rarely located in one place; however, coordination between those specialists is critical and should be done when a patient is brought in for consultation. Just as your cardiology consultant will coordinate among medical management—interventional cardiologists and surgical colleagues—cancer pain treatment often, but not always, has matured to the point where such interprovider specialist consultation occurs.

From the perspective of survivorship, for those patients with progressive cancer, continuity of care is more perfected than for patients who have a good treatment response. Ironically, with the relief of a good response, patients often reduce doses of medications on a self-determined schedule, and that is often too quickly. Most patients suffer for a few days; a few wind up needing emergency department care in an acute withdrawal. So, many patients and their families are relieved to be off medications that practically and emotionally tether them to the cancer treatment they would like to put behind that they are willing to endure the discomfort, no matter how severe and transient. A few even see it as a rite of passage. The symptoms of a *mini-withdrawal* can be avoided.

Ongoing Pain Assessment

Beyond the scope of the NCCN guidelines, various subsyndromal pain syndromes extend after treatment is over. Their nature pertains to the type of cancer a patient had and type of treatment a patient received. Ongoing and often overlooked pain issues include:

Breast cancer: neuropathic pain at the surgical scar, bone pain

Colon cancer: pain at colostomy site

Rectal cancer: neuropathic and pressure pain when seated and with each bowel movement

Prostate cancer: urination pain, bone pain

Lung cancer (also esophageal, mediastinal lymphoma, or thymoma): pain on swallowing, indigestion, inspiratory pain caused by fibrosis, reduced volume

CNS cancers: deficits at the areas controlled by the tissues at the treated site

Cervical, vulvar cancers: dyspareunia, severe dryness

Head and neck cancers: xerostomia or mucositis, dysgeusia, pain when talking or swallowing, osteoradionecrosis of the jaw, ear pain

Common treatment-related etiologies include neuropathic pain after chemotherapies, particularly of the vinca alkaloid, taxane and platinum families; neuropathic pain as a result of inevitable postoperative nerve compromise; fibrosis of previously pliable tissues after radiation therapy; and *radiation recall* after platinum-, methotrexate-, doxorubicin-, dactinomycin-, or taxane-based regimen. It is tempting to believe that the pain will diminish over time, but for some patients, the pain syndromes become chronic, needing chronic treatment. A minority of patients *without a precancer history of substance use or dependence* remain on opioids for a long time, perhaps for the rest of their lives. A general strategy for patients who are left with residual pain is to maximize—to the fullest extent possible—treatment with adjuvant, nonopioid analgesics, nonpharmacologic treatments, and anesthetic procedures wherever feasible and effective. Although noncancer patients have been maintained on opioids for many years via methadone maintenance programs, we are only just getting to know the consequences of long-term opioid use, such as secondary hypogonadism.

The NCCN Adult Pain Guidelines enumerate nonpharmacological treatments useful in cancer pain management that include massage, transcutaneous electrical nerve stimulation (TENS) units, physical therapy, acupuncture or acupressure, and ultrasound, as well as many types of cognitive therapies such as relaxation, distraction, imagery, hypnosis, and spiritual care. Find reliable providers where you practice.

General Opioid Tapering Guidelines

Apart from knowing which practitioners in your community can help with the non-pharmacologic treatments, the initial tapering often falls to the cancer specialist, and mostly without warning during a follow-up visit. Patients and families often initiate tapering too quickly on their own for fear they will be on opioids for life. Some overall principles include the following:

- Establish actual regular usage in 24 hours. Add up all fixed doses used and any *prn* (as needed) doses used. Use the commonly available tables (NCCN guidelines contain easy to use tables).
- Temporarily convert short-acting formulations to long-acting versions of the closest related opioid with the goal of then tapering. Using the long-acting preparations will avoid miniwithdrawals between doses. (Continuous release preparations of oxycodone, morphine, or hydromorphone; transdermal preparations of fentanyl or methadone are likely candidates.)
- If long-acting preparations are not available (it is common for pharmacies in high crime areas to avoid stocking long-acting opioids) through prescription plan or carry a cumbersome co-pay, use the short-acting preparation on a fixed schedule *every 3 hours*, limiting to only one middle-of-the-night dose, if possible, to avoid further interrupting sleep. If the patient is an inpatient or in a facility, be sure to write the order as *around the clock while awake* so that the dose missed because of sleep can be given upon awakening if the patient is not yet due for the next dose.
- Once on a stable dose, reduce the dose *slowly*. How slowly depends on *how long* the patient has been on opioids and their precancer use. The *fastest* taper should be *no quicker than* 50% of the dose every 3 days *on a fixed-dose schedule*, and most schedules should be accomplished much more slowly. Reductions of 5% a week for patients who have been on long-term opioid use take both persistence and patience.

- At these low doses, referral to substance abuse experts is often not helpful as they are used to dealing with patients on much higher doses and are less experienced with the treatment of chronic nausea post-cancer treatment. Substituting other agents is key in helping the program be successful.
- Using medications as adjuvants to minimize withdrawal at the end of the tapering period can be helpful. Antihistamines such as scopolamine (TranScop® and others) changed every 3 days, used behind the ear on alternating sides or low doses of a long-acting benzodiazepine *for a few (5–10) days (e.g., clonazepam 0.25 or 0.5 mg bid or tid)* at the end of the tapering period can help the uneasiness that occurs during that final period. Longer periods of benzodiazepine use add only sedation without analgesia.
- Refer for nonpharmacologic approaches: relaxation training, diversionary activities when available.
- The most successful tapering plans are often the slowest because the patient's optimism and adherence are strongest on the first try.
- Once the very last dose is reached, a small supply (10 doses, for instance) of the short-acting equivalent can be helpful for the patient to have at home and to use on a *prn* basis to reduce the last vestiges of abdominal cramping and diarrhea.

▨ BENZODIAZEPINE TAPERING

Benzodiazepine tapering uses the same principles. Patients have often been taking benzodiazepines for weeks or months as an antiemetic during chemotherapy and radiation therapy, for sleep afterward or as an anxiolytic. Patients often "run out" of their prescription and do not realize that tapering is necessary to avoid withdrawal. Many times, a visit to an urgent care center or emergency department is made for a routine chief complaint of being "nauseous after chemotherapy" or being "nauseous after radiation therapy," and the result in a *stat* dose of lorazepam and prescriptions for it with another antiemetic. Compounding the situation is the simultaneous use of *nonbenzodiazepine* sleep medicines that also come with cross-tolerance and dependence and a withdrawal that looks just like benzodiazepine withdrawal.

A plan to withdraw the benzodiazepine slowly and use alternate antiemetics is often the most successful approach. If patients have used benzodiazepines "for years" as a sedative-hypnotic or anxiolytic, the time for tapering needs to be extended and can be months.

The approach is often the same for opioids:

- Establish actual regular usage in 24 hours. Add up all fixed doses used and any *prn* doses used.
- Temporarily convert short-acting formulations to long-acting versions of the closest related opioid with the goal of then tapering. Using the long-acting preparations will avoid miniwithdrawals between doses. Long-acting benzodiazepines like clonazepam (Klonopin® and others) or slow-release preparations of diazepam or alprazolam are helpful.

- Reduce the long-acting preparation on a *fixed dose schedule*, reducing by 50% every 5 days at the quickest; it is often best to use a smaller reduction over more days.
- When a patient remains symptomatic during the taper, and is well after the acute and early delayed phases of emesis during chemotherapy, the usual 5-HT$_3$ blockers are not helpful or not approved for reimbursement by prescription plans. Alternatives, and the more effective medications for chronic, low-level nausea are antihistamines, such as scopolamine in a transdermal patch (TranScop® and others), changed every 3 days, used behind the ear on alternating sides or diphenhydramine (Benadryl® and others). Diphenhydramine is the most widely used antihistamine as an antiemetic, is sedating, and may cause urinary hesitancy or, rarely, retention in men with enlarged prostates. Women with stress incontinence sometimes get some relief for two problems with one medication. A second good alternative is dronabinol (Marinol® and others) or nabilone (Cesamet® and others), cannabinoids congeners offering good relief from chronic, low-level nausea posttreatment. Although there is some withdrawal from cannabinoids as well, it is less uncomfortable because its use will only be a few weeks to relieve the vestiges of nausea. Patients who have used much recreational marijuana over the course of their lives may need higher than the usual doses (up to 2.5–10 mg tid of dronabinol; up to 1–2 mg bid for nabilone). Potent ginger supplements (rather than ginger ale or cookies) are available in many health food stores and can also be a great help.
- Nonpharmacologic approaches: relaxation training and diversions can be of great help. If indeed an underlying anxiety problem has been treated with the antiemetics, referral to a behavioral health specialist with cancer experience is warranted.
- As with opioids, the most successful tapering plans are often the slowest because the patient's enthusiasm peaks on the first try.

▒ DYSPNEA

Dyspnea is a common symptom treated regularly in any primary care practice, with both cardiac and pulmonary etiologies. Patients with chronic obstructive pulmonary disease (COPD) as those with cancer have benefited from the explosion in medical and pharmacologic technology with ever smaller devices that concentrate oxygen allowing greater mobility, drugs, and drug delivery that reduces the inflammatory component.

The treatment of asthma has also improved with matching advances in pharmacology and ambulatory oxygen supplementation.

Dyspnea is of special note in cancer survivors as a symptom needing attention because of the lengthened period of survival. After treatment, patients do often experience shortness of breath from cancer, residual from cancer therapy, or because of preexisting pulmonary or cardiac disease such as COPD, congestive heart failure, nonmalignant pleural effusion, inflammatory pneumonitis, or bronchospasm associated with asthma. Fatigue or significant weight change can worsen breathlessness. Often, the cause is multifactored.

Treatment should first target relief of the cancer with the traditional modalities. Correction of fatigue and cachexia or weight gain, where possible, is also important.

Symptomatic relief should *not* be limited to end-of-life care alone. Applying the same techniques during long-term survivorship as that period is much longer than previously experienced. A concise review by Dy and colleagues[18] summarizes evidence-based care. Traditionally, morphine has been used to relieve dyspnea during end-of-life care, and when the dose is titrated and used judiciously, it is helpful during the period of survivorship not simply in the last stages. Being marketed in tablets, quick-dissolve tablets, liquid, long-acting tablets, and in a parenteral form that can be used intravenously or subcutaneously, morphine dosing can be tailored to suit clinical needs. Nebulized preparations have not been found effective. Other treatments that have been found effective include oxygen therapy and beta-agonists for the obstructive component.

Treatment of malignant pleural effusion is important as a cause of dyspnea for both survival and quality of life. This can be accomplished by bedside chest tube or an ambulatory Pleurx® catheter. In a randomized trial conducted by the Cancer and Leukemia Group B, a quality of life (QOL) advantage was found with equal mortality and increased morbidity of a minimally invasive insufflation with talc installation done in the operating room compared to a bedside chest tube. Patients reported that they were more comfortable, felt safer, and had better control of their pain coupled with a decrease in fatigue. Improved pain control for Pleurx® is owed to heightened post-op vigilance over routine provision of analgesia at the bedside.[19]

With little work done to investigate the evidence basis of other treatments, patients who have fibrosis from radiation therapy or restrictive lung disease from certain agents such as bleomycin, application of the treatments used in noncancer COPD, asthma, and congestive heart failure (CHF) are often used. Pulmonary rehabilitation during the preoperative, perioperative, and postoperative periods can be quite helpful as an adjunct to medical management.[20]

The important message in the treatment of dyspnea in cancer survivors is to incorporate both of what is best from end-of-life care *and* treatments used in COPD and CHF in a noncancer population. With a lack of evidence-based treatments for any one particular symptom, we should not neglect noncancer pulmonary therapies and should also consider morphine, even though it has been pigeon-holed by some clinicians for the end of life. Ipatropium/albuterol inhalers or hand-held nebulizers or inhaled steroids can be of great relief although not fully tested. Using a fan to move air around and over a desk or bed or in a room can also help greatly. Aminophylline, theophylline, and caffeine can also help clear airways, although their use in COPD and asthma has waned. Corticosteroids are often used, with good effect and little clinical evidence. Management of secretions, liquefying with guaifenesin over-the-counter preparations or drying with antihistamines or any other anticholinergic drug can also offer comfort and relief of dyspnea.

■ ALCOHOL DEPENDENCE AND CANCER

Ethanol-containing products, mostly consumed for recreational purposes, are a "multiedged" sword in the development of cancer and the struggle to maintain a cancer-free survival. Apart from the usual effects in the general population on the liver, brain, heart, bones, and practically every other organ system, alcohol's promotion of oncogenesis for initial cancers or recurrences is virtually beyond dispute. Whether through chronic inflammation, the interference or promotion of metabolic pathways, or central effects that ease our avoidance of risky behaviors, alcohol in more than minimal quantities is a public health threat. Specifically in cancer, regular heavy alcohol consumption is implicated to cause cancers of the liver, esophagus, larynx, pharynx, and oral cavity and increase the risks for the aerodigestive cancers. Moderate use among women has been related with increases in breast cancer, and prostate cancer in men.[21] Although the beneficial effects of tannins and other compounds in red wines such as resveratrol are likely of health benefit, their benefit is in doses that the body can extract from the wine itself. They can be consumed in other products avoiding the deleterious effects of the alcohol that is paired with them.

A Watershed Moment

The question requiring sound clinical judgment comes when a patient with anything more than occasional alcohol use is diagnosed with cancer. Knowing the emotional turmoil of that experience, the wisdom of using the diagnosis as a *teachable moment* has its advantages and disadvantages. Although the scare of the diagnosis may provide the additional kick to one's motivation to carefully taper or stop drinking alcohol-containing products, such a watershed moment may work for some patients, but not all. It is possible or even likely that attempts have been made in the past to taper or stop but have not been successful because of the addictive properties of alcohol. The "feel good" effects of alcohol may be a distinct component of coping with a life-threatening diagnosis and harder to give up at a time of great distress.

The detoxification and relapse prevention of the use of alcoholic beverages is somewhat divorced from the world of oncology treatment. However, because of the complexities and time a successful detox and time-proven sobriety take, referral to cancer-sensitive programs or clinicians is essential. Except in extraordinary circumstances, detoxification is not feasible in one or two office visits or while the patient is admitted to the hospital—unless there is concomitant care from a substance abuse specialist. The type of confrontation and honesty of reporting to the substance abuse provider is different from what is practiced, in general, in oncology. There is also a divergence in the underlying theoretical framework of treatment between those who believe that complete abstinence is optimal and those who accept an occasional slip. One of the most successful maintenance approaches for sobriety—known worldwide as "AA" or *Alcoholics Anonymous*—has irregularly welcomed cancer patients who use "psychoactive substances" such as opioids for cancer pain or benzodiazepines or cannabinoids as antiemetics. Although AA would not support a specialty chapter run out of a cancer center as recently as 2008,* luckily, patients in many parts of the country

---

*Personally experienced in my role as director of Cancer Supportive Services at Continuum Cancer Centers of New York when attempting to cosponsor an existing AA group for patients with cancer where prescription opioids and benzodiazepines with the explicit use for pain or nausea are monitored

do report an informal practice where there is an existing member of a chapter who is a cancer survivor and is a willing *sponsor* of a patient in treatment. Thus, allowances are made for professionally prescribed opioids or benzodiazepines when clear-cut agreements with the provider are in place.

Referral to a substance abuse specialist will also help the oncology team to decide if a patient needs a formal, medically supervised detoxification program, whether inpatient or outpatient, that prescribes sedatives over a few days to minimize *delirium tremens* and prophylaxis against withdrawal seizures also involves the patient in a community of others for mutual support. Just as much chemotherapy is administered as an outpatient, some detox programs are also outpatient programs, under the same cost-saving pressures to responsibly spend our health care dollars. Sobriety maintenance has evolved after many years of AA experience to offer an interpersonal safety net when temptations occur. Coordinating a mandatory daily substance abuse visit, regularly scheduled daily radiation therapy visits, and time-sensitive chemotherapy sessions is possible but quite difficult.

Importance of the Oncology Team's Role

The
LEARN
System©

p. 138
Important
Revelations
to My
Treatment
Team

In a way that is direct, honest, and (not too) scary but factual, the oncology team needs to *triage* the amount of alcohol actually used to get the right patients to the right programs locally. That begins with the screening you and your staff do on consultation. Just as we have learned the right way to collect a history about sexual practices to screen for HIV and other sexually transmitted diseases that are critical comorbidities during cancer treatment—asking the "right" questions is vital. You will develop your own words and approach; however, certain talking points must be kept in mind. The *Important Revelations to My Treatment Team* may help quantify current usage and open up the dialogue, but not serve as a replacement for the vital interaction.

- Everyone's idea of *social drinking* is vastly different. Using that term in the *Social History* helps no one. Ask specifically, "On a daily or weekly basis, how many 1 oz servings of hard liquor (e.g., vodka, gin, scotch) or 6 oz servings of wine or 8 oz servings of beer do you consume regularly? If not regularly, *how often?*"
- Emphasize with the maximal amount of *gravitas* and *alarm* you can muster how alcohol dependence can interfere with successful cancer treatment: from truly understanding informed consent to the metabolic changes while administering chemotherapy and radiation therapy that makes it hard to manage the cancer treatment (liver function, esophagitis, worsened neuropathy), to the virtual undoing of hard treatment through continual chronic inflammation by promoting recurrence.
- If the patient is actively drinking to the point where you question the ability to consent or if he or she arrives so intoxicated that aspiration is a risk, affirm that chemotherapy or radiation therapy will not be given that day, and if the patient presents for treatment inebriated, you will insist comanagement with a substance abuse expert.

If you practice in a larger center, involve the social worker, chaplain, and mental health services as well as the patient navigator; especially include the patient's family (with Health Insurance Portability and Accountability Act [HIPAA] consent, of course).

▧ NICOTINE DEPENDENCE

Virtually, everything that you do in the face of alcohol dependence is mirrored in your place in nicotine dependence, with minor difference. Although specialty programs exist throughout the country—from community-based abstinence programs to inpatient units for recidivist smokers—much of nicotine withdrawal takes place in the primary care provider's office.

Important clinical points include the following:

- Ascertain *exactly* how much nicotine-containing products a patient uses or second-hand exposure to tobacco smoke: cigarettes smoked (in whole or in part), chewing tobacco, cigars and exposure to second-hand smoke in the workplace or recreationally. (Visit a casino, in most locations, to estimate the amount of second-hand smoke exposure one can receive passively and innocently.)
- With the proper amount of *gravitas* and *alarm*, emphasize the negative effects of tobacco smoke on remaining cancer-free and how stopping is essential. If a patient has end-stage cancer at diagnosis where the life expectancy is days or weeks, many colleagues would take the exact opposite approach and avoid having a patient spend sparse energy on being nicotine-, smoke-, or tobacco-free, except where supplemental oxygen is used. Hospitals vary by locale and philosophy about having areas where patients may smoke. If by local ordinance or hospital policy, no smoking is allowed, or a patient is in a critical care unit or nonambulatory even with assistance, make sure to provide nicotine replacement via transdermal patch to avoid acute withdrawal, which will not only be uncomfortable, but will also affect drug metabolism through abrupt cessation.
- Be extremely careful not to *blame* a patient who has developed a cancer where tobacco products are implicated. Knowing the allegations of product design where the most dependence-producing forms of nicotine were used in tobacco production and the societal acceptance in the 1940s and 1950s through the early 1960s—be empathic and firm.
- Wherever possible, providers staff, and often oncology nurses will seize a *teachable moment* to educate family members of the risks of second-hand smoke.
- For disease-free survivors ending or after treatment, strongly encourage enrolling in a smoke-enders program in your area.
- Be familiar with the various forms of nicotine replacement (transdermal patches in various strengths, nicotine gum, nose sprays) and the two prescription drugs approved to minimize nicotine withdrawal cravings: varenicline (Chantix® and others) and bupropion (Zyban® and others). These and a variety of antidepressants decrease the central component of craving. Caution should be used in

prescriptions during chemotherapy (possible interaction with taxanes or anti-emetics). The pharmacologic principle is to reduce cravings and substitute nicotine unbound to the dangerous impurities in tobacco help someone cut down and stop the offending product. Then, step down the nicotine slowly to avoid withdrawal. These techniques are most successful when tied to a behavioral program that attacks the habitual aspects of smoking. When a person smokes, what are the triggers, what to do with your hands, avoiding weight changes—these are vital components that require attention to avoid relapse.

- Relocate any smokers' area *away from* entrances to your offices or cancer centers to avoid patients and families seeing trusted staff members smoking as they come for appointments or treatment. Offer incentives to *all staff* to quit nicotine and tobacco products—even if that means time off to attend a local program—and coverage for nicotine replacement or crave-reducing medications, which sometimes have limited or no reimbursement.

- Know which programs are in your area, if your cancer center, general hospital, American Cancer Society office, or chapter of the American Lung Association runs or has access to programs. Individual houses of worship may have the programs as well.

5

Easing Communication in Multiprovider Management

▨ COMMUNICATION WITH COLLEAGUES

Effective communication *should* be easier with today's technological advances, but it seems as if it has gotten more complicated and harder. Some of us still work from paper charts, some have moved into the electronic medical record, and some are in hybrid mode as the transition occurs. Privacy and confidentiality policies make it risky to send health information over the Internet and do not allow practitioners without local privileges access to proprietary networks. When patients are treated locally within a small system by providers who see each other regularly, much communication happens informally, for instance, in the parking lot or before or after meetings. With further subspecialization and centers of excellence outside of the local hospital or multispecialty practice, the informal mechanism no longer suffices and the formal mechanisms are still not accessible to all.

Communication between primary care providers (PCPs) and oncology specialists is most effective when it is timely and targeted. The referring provider needs to know that a patient did follow through with the consultation, and what the resulting opinions of the consultant are. Much interchange during treatment optimizes the coordination of care. At the completion of treatment, an effective and seamless handoff from one provider to the other can take place as expectations about surveillance and late treatment effects can be passed between providers.

Varying treatment systems and reimbursement systems affect the way we move our patients through diagnosis, treatment, and follow-up. How we communicate with colleagues depends on many factors, including how patient responsibilities are shared at various points: during the work-up and during treatment—especially when patients switch treatment modalities, immediately after treatment, and during extended survival. The division of labor delineating which provider will handle the evaluation and treatment of comorbidities will also determine how communication will occur. Maintain referrals with a simple principle, "Do Good Work. Be Nice. Build Trust."[22]

Work-Ups and Initial Consultation

Most work-ups for cancer that begin with a suspicious lump, an unexpected finding on an imaging studies, excessive unintended weight loss, or fatigue are done in the primary care setting. Unexpected anemia, thrombocytopenia or neutropenia are often discovered by chance on routine examination. A persistent lump may be referred to a general surgical colleague or in some settings, to an interventional radiologist. Breast lesions tend to get referred directly to breast surgeons, skin lesions to a dermatologist, and unexpected vaginal bleeding directly to gynecologists. Regional CT scans are often done by the PCP as well.

Communication Strategies at Consultation and Throughout Treatment

At Consult, for the Referring Provider

Call the consultant and quickly summarize what you have found, including any important comorbidities that the consultant should know about. Share expectations of transferred care, or comanagement. Offer to be of help. Being diplomatically explicit to indicate whether you will expect to see the patient during or after treatment can help avoid later misunderstanding.

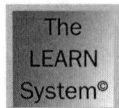

The LEARN System©

p. 133
What Is
Important
to Me

Follow up the call with a brief referral note that outlines a current problem list, pertinent past history, and current medication list. Restate your intentions about follow-up you mentioned on the telephone. Include copies of pathology reports, imaging, and blood work to serve as a baseline, unless these are available on a shared data system. *What Is Important to Me* has information usable to both the PCP and the cancer team, so it should also be appended.

At Consult, for the Oncology Specialist

In return, a short telephone call summarizing your findings and the initial plan of care will probably be greatly appreciated. It allays the fear that once a patient is referred, he or she is "lost to follow-up," particularly if the referring provider is at a tertiary care facility located down the road or in a neighboring city. Any immediate comanagement coordination can be discussed. Also, follow up the call with a consultation note that mentions the phone call and gives more detail about the initial treatment to the extent it is known. If the work-up lacks certain elements, advise the referring provider of what's needed so he or she may offer authorization if necessitated by the insurance carrier, or follow through with the missing elements, and make sure to copy the referring provider for informational and educational purposes. Supplying the electronic link to the *NCCN Guidelines* if that is what your cancer center uses can also help the PCP see that a national standard is being addressed, even as deviations from the guidelines tailor the treatment to individual needs. If you have the computer skills, print out the schema, or in an electronic record, even better to append the guideline file as a "pdf" to your note.

Depending on how your practice is structured, a call should be made to the patient or family from the referring provider or office staff to confirm that the initial contact was made. In a well-tuned system, your office manager or nurse can make that call when the chart is put together or make a routine call the next working day if the process is electronic.

During Treatment

Communication Strategy

A hospitalist team often manages inpatients while in the hospital, adding an additional set of providers to the communication matrix. Without a unified electronic record system, it is unlikely that the referring provider and the oncologist's consult note will arrive on the chart soon enough to avoid duplicating tests that have been done in the ambulatory setting. A call to the hospitalist team may help, and sending the notes to the hospital unit by fax may be the only solution if an e-mail with the documents attached is not secure. If admission is through the emergency department, another set of providers may need a quick interim summary from you if they too are not on the same electronic system.

▨ USE *MY RECOVERY PLAN* TO FOSTER EFFECTIVE COMMUNICATION

The *Communicator Sheets* in *My Recovery Plan* can help ease this burden. Information that needs to be passed between providers is summarized on this form that can be given to the patient or family who should show it to both the emergency department and hospitalist teams. A thought-provoking debate about how much responsibility should be given to the patient and family is interesting to undertake at conferences or departmental meetings, but for efficiency and ease, it is the most direct process that compensates for the absence of a unified electronic record. A copy can be forwarded to the referring PCP as well to fill the gap that often occurs with the PCP more involved during the work-up and after treatment rather than in between. Patients and families should carry back the updated information and any other pertinent lab or imaging reports for the PCP and managing oncologists who may not be able to access notes from the emergency department or hospitalist.

Cancer subspecialists differ somewhat in the timing of pivotal communications when not on a shared information system. Radiation oncologists will usually send an Initial Consultation Note and a Treatment Summary after the first off-treatment visit is complete. Surgical oncologists often send a Consult Note and then a Final Summary Note with a copy of the Operative Note. Medical oncologists send a Consultation Note and, less often, a summary upon completion of treatment. Other specialists (pain management, nutritional support, genetics, physical medicine and rehabilitation, counseling providers) would be best copying their notes to all of the cancer specialists because the provider doing on-going care and follow-up can vary so widely. If a patient is referred to a particular investigator to assess eligibility for a clinical trial, yet another group of providers needs access to the same information, requiring another vital duplication of the information. A duplicative phone call may be necessary along with forwarding documents. The advent of common unified electronic record systems should greatly reduce the effort to pass information back and forth via mail and fax, but only a few networks are set up thus far.

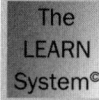

The
LEARN
System©

p. 143-150
My Recovery
Plan
Communicator

The
LEARN
System©

p. 141
My Weekly
Recovery
Planner

Communication for Cancer-Related Emergencies

Divergent patterns of care and challenges in communication affect how cancer-related emergencies are handled. Commonly, these involve cord compression, hypercalcemia, tumor lysis syndrome, superior vena cava syndrome, febrile neutropenia, or pericardial tamponade. Fever over a threshold defined by the managing oncologist, an unexpected change in mental status, or hemorrhage may need emergency evaluation.

In virtually all treatment settings, most of these bona fide emergencies will require emergency admission. Patients or families may call the referring provider or any of the cancer subspecialists with an worrisome symptom, and in general, the subspecialist who is giving the most prominent treatment of the moment is the likely recipient of the phone call. Patients involved in concomitant radiation therapy and chemotherapy treatments may call either or both. The less threatening symptoms, such as a subtle change in mental status or fatigue that develops within hours, can result in home management, such as an increase in oral hydration, oral antibiotics, and an office visit should be made on the next working day after suggestions can be made on the telephone. Because a scheduled radiation treatment or infusion may be out of the question for the next day, formal notification to the other team providers needs to take place. A chance hallway meeting will not suffice. Unified electronic records often have a feature that alerts any current provider about a hospital or emergency department admission that has occurred on sign in. Duplicating that information exchange manually is the bane of on-call decision making, with the extra burden of cross notification. Providers new to the community or network can solidify their reputations by communicating well among stakeholders.

Communication at Follow-up and Survivorship Care Remain the Biggest Challenge

Information exchange becomes more of a challenge after treatment ends. The transfer of information to community providers has become a more formidable task with treatments becoming more complicated and an increased period of survivorship. The Institute of Medicine report, *From Cancer Patient to Cancer Survivor: Lost in Transition*, proposes the adoption of survivorship care reports.[1a] Use of survivorship care reports can circumvent many of the obstacles in passing clinical information to future providers. Survivorship plans vary in content, with standardized plans available through American Society of Clinical Oncology (ASCO)[23] and in *Journey Forward*, a collaborative effort of the National Coalition of Cancer Survivorship, the University of California, Los Angeles (UCLA) Cancer Survivorship Center, the insurance carrier Wellpoint, and Genentech.[24] A user-friendly guide, including a survivorship care plan builder on CD or downloadable online, is available so that plans for breast and colon cancer, lymphoma, and a general template can be used to incorporate survivorship plans into daily practice. Personal Health Records for many of the major cancer sites are featured in this book.

Completing the document can be either a simple or onerous task that can be shared by patients and staff. Hahn and Ganz[25] have piloted selected approaches in different treatment settings: an academic cancer center, community hospital, county hospital, and primary care medical group. The plans were completed with the combined efforts of staff and patients, and the patient and providers retained copies on paper or a scanned electronic version, in the primary care practice. They concluded that the design and implementation of survivorship plans will vary by setting and "one size does not fit all."

Communication About the Future: Developing and Evaluating a Survivorship Plan

In response to the IOM Report, along with colleagues at the Continuum Cancer Centers of New York, we developed and completed a pilot study to evaluate a survivorship plan for patients with head and neck cancers. With programs underway focusing on survivorship plans for a variety of other solid tumors, and with a large patient base of head and neck cancer patients at our location, the New York Community Trust funded the program, under the direction of Ronald Blum MD to both meet a specific need and to add to the experience in the field. With a multidisciplinary staff and input from patient volunteers, we compiled a compact *Personal Health Record* (*PHR*) that was given to patients at the end of their treatment, and offered it on paper and on flash (thumb) drive in an electronic version. An evaluation component was built into the study, using the FACT-H&N, a specially made *Satisfaction with Survivorship Care Plan* assessment. A subset of family caregivers was asked to complete a *Brief Assessment Scale for Caregiver Burden*. In the small sample, patients were satisfied with the PHR Survivorship Plan on paper and electronically. The family members felt too overburdened to complete the assessments. Pilot studies such as this one can provide valuable information for program development. For example, the patients assessed were fatigued and uncomfortable with stomatitis and excess secretions, and they were too distressed to focus on the need they would have for portable documentation in the future. Completion of the PHR in the absence of a unified electronic medical record proved timely but possible. But once the severe side effects of treatment began to wane, patients and families appreciated the PHRs for communicating with outside providers. A copy of the abstract submitted is in Figure 1 on the next page.

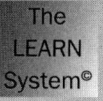

The LEARN System©

p. 168
Your Personal Health Record

■ PERSONAL HEALTH RECORDS CAN ALSO STRESS PATIENT/CAREGIVER RESPONSIBILITIES

Most versions of survivorship plans available have many common data points, summarizing type and stage of cancer, type of treatment, possible late effects, and surveillance. This important, basic information can be augmented with some additional information usable by the patient and the family *at the time they receive the survivorship plan*. The *Personal Health Records* featured in this book—in *My Recovery Plan*—include information about *what patients need to do right away* and can be adapted from The LEARN System.

■ YOUR ENDORSEMENT IS CRITICAL

As with other health maintenance advice, a provider's clear direction is essential to stress the importance on the self-administered dimensions of *Activity, Rest, and Nutrition*.

Background: A 2006 Institute of Medicine report, *From Cancer Patient to Cancer Survivor: Lost in Transition*, found gaps in communication, inattention to long- and short-term sequelae of treatment, and lack of guidance posttreatment. This pilot developed, implemented, and evaluated a Personal Health Record (PHR) for head and neck cancer survivors (HNCS) consisting of a comprehensive care summary and individualized follow-up plan to bridge those gaps, address multiple posttreatment needs, and improve health and quality of life (QOL).

Methods: Prospective 1-year study of 100 HNCS without recurrence at 6 months, age 29 to 86 years (mean 57.5 years). The PHR included demographics, diagnostics, treatment summaries, follow-up, prevention, and counseling information. QOL was assessed at baseline (N = 95), 6 months (N = 53) and 1 year (N = 33) using the FACT-H&N. A 10 patient subset completed a brief assessment scale for caregiver burden and satisfaction with survivorship care plan survey. All patients received a PHR on paper and 96 on a 1 GB flash drive as a record for community-based providers. We examined barriers to implementation.

Results: Statistically significant improvements were shown in overall QOL, physical well-being, functional well-being, and items specific to HNCS: dry mouth, swallowing, eating solid foods, and communicating, all likely resulting from the healing process. Social and emotional well-being remained stable. HNCS (n = 9) were very satisfied or satisfied with the PHR. Caregiver distress could not be measured as many patients came without a caregiver and others felt too overwhelmed to complete the questionnaire. The next step is to overcome barriers to implementation and integration into clinical practice, including synthesizing treatment data from disparate charts into a unified PHR in the absence of uniform electronic health records.

Conclusions: (1) It is feasible to provide a paper or electronic PHR posttreatment. (2) The PHR empowers patients and facilitates communication and awareness of treatment sequelae and responsibility for transition to survivorship in multimodal complex treatment of HNC. (3) Patients were satisfied with the PHR although sample size was small.

ASCO Meeting Abstracts Jun 9, 2011:e19514

FIGURE 5.1 Feasibility of implementing a personalized electronic health record for head and neck cancer patients.
S. B. Fleishman, M. Bookbinder, E. Silen, B. Buddhdev, S. Shah, P. Homel, J. Nabatian, V. Rosenwald, R. H. Blum, funded by the New York Community Trust; Continuum Cancer Centers of New York: Beth Israel, New York, NY

In your own words, emphasize that a commitment to a survivorship program needs to be more sustaining than a New Year's resolution or a fleeting self-promise. Reiterate the overlap to heart-healthy living recommendations and how they are virtually the same.

DISTRIBUTION OF THE PERSONAL HEALTH RECORD

Patients lighten the burden of consent and transmission when they personally give their PHR disc to be downloaded into other providers' electronic charts, or submit a paper copy. Patient-centered distribution also makes it a dynamic system. For example, when a patient moves or changes jobs, it often provokes a change in providers, and the patient can bring the necessary information to his or her provider or send it in advance of his or her office visit.

YOUR ROLE IN EDUCATING PRIMARY CARE PROVIDERS WHO PROVIDE ONGOING CARE

Completing the communication loop with the PCP who will be again assuming responsibilities for much of the follow-up will help everyone. It will supply the information that most PCPs need, and very much want, and imprint your "brand" in their practices to encourage future referrals. In a 2009 Editorial in the *Journal of Clinical Oncology*, Nekhlyudov[26] nicely summarizes that PCPs want basic education, guidance, and familiarity with local resources in the following areas:

- cancer surveillance modalities, intervals, and duration
- guidelines for general and risk-based screening for other cancers
- surveillance for and management of treatment-related morbidity, including potential
- interactions between cancer and noncancer medications or treatment prevention and risk-modifying strategies such as diet and exercise
- counseling for genetic implications for patients and their families
- resources for possible financial and other psychosocial implications of cancer or treatment
- coordination of care, if needed, with whom, and when

WILL FUTURE PREDICTED SHORTAGES IN THE ONCOLOGY WORKFORCE MOVE SURVIVORSHIP CARE TO NON-ONCOLOGISTS?

In 2009, Shulman and colleagues[27] forecast that shortages in the number of oncology and primary care providers in the workforce will decrease more than originally calculated, coincident with the complexity of care and the increasing numbers of survivors.

One of the suggestions they propose is for nurse practitioners or physician assistants who work cooperatively with the oncologist and see patients for routine follow-up visits, and that part of the time at the end of treatment can be used to develop and discuss a survivorship plan that is guideline-based and linked to quality-of-care measures similar to what is used for patients with diabetes and heart disease. With the potential shortages in the primary care specialties as well, they propose that a new cadre of nurse practitioners and physician assistants may collaborate with oncology subspecialists to help manage the growing survivor population.

6

Effectively Managing the Transitional Points in Care

▦ WHEN THE NEWS IS GOOD

Good news is easy to report. Patients who *don't* have cancer rarely make their way to medical or radiation oncology practices (hematology patients excepted). Surgical oncologists can sometimes, after preparing a patient and family for a diagnosis of cancer, find that a tumor is benign. Most of the time, that news is imparted cheerfully and with a great sense of relief. The patient is usually seen through the postoperative recovery period and then referred back to the referring provider if not co-managed through the surgical admission. From the provider's perspective, such rewarding encounters provide a welcome interlude to the more frequent scenario of being the first to confirm a cancer diagnosis to concerned patient and family. That news is actually shrouded in uncertainty, and a final pathology report is necessary to confirm clinical suspicion.

Medical and radiation oncologists can also bear good news with a good response to treatment. These encounters are similarly colored by a degree of uncertainty because often, but not always, cancer may be slowly reappearing somewhere, too small to detect at that moment, but able to show itself in the future. Such good news moments give everyone something to celebrate and a time to show gratitude.

In keeping with the theme of healing and health maintenance, these are also golden opportunities to reinforce the proactive elements of The LEARN System. The debate continues about the effectiveness of practitioners' reminders to lose weight, stop using tobacco products, exercise more, and drink less alcohol to actually influence adherence. Such advice during routine office visits may or may not effect a sustained change in health behavior. A *halo effect* from the report of good news may leverage rejoicing into a teachable moment. It could just be the right moment. Using the staged model of smoking cessation,[28] this can be the ideal time to move a patient through precontemplation to contemplation, preparation and action using The LEARN System. Good opportunities do not come often enough.

▦ WHEN THE NEWS IS BAD

The basic principles of SPIKES (*s*et up, *p*erception, *i*nvite response, *k*nowledge, *e*xplore) can be adapted to delivering difficult news at patient visits. Although each one has some idiosyncrasies of the moment, there is a set of common skills that can easily be adopted. When a full SPIKES-inspired discussion is too cumbersome for the circumstances, there are three basic steps to follow. Throughout practice, I have adapted a system based on what I had learned at certificate program at the Center for Creative Leadership[29] in Greensboro, North Carolina: **<u>a</u>ssess**, **<u>c</u>onvey**, and **<u>s</u>upport**, an easy-to-remember acronym because it is one we commonly use as an abbreviation for the American Cancer Society.

Here are some instances when these three simple-to-remember prompts can guide the difficult conversations and make communication easier and more effective at these predictable transition points in care:

- Discussing a suspicious symptom and need for further testing
- Revealing a diagnosis (use SPIKES)
- Introducing the role of clinical trials
- Starting and stopping each modality
- Paradoxical distress at the end of treatment (radiation therapy in particular)
- Revealing a recurrence or relapse
- Introducing palliative care and hospice

Discussing a Suspicious Symptom and Need for Further Testing

Although this task often falls to primary care providers and surgical oncologists, medical and radiation oncologists will find it helpful during treatment when a suspicious symptom occurs such as bone pain or explosive diarrhea. One could think of many examples where it could be used.

> <u>Patient</u> (64-year-old man being treated for prostate cancer with external beam RT): I was getting up from a chair, and I don't remember twisting but I suddenly got a really bad pain in my back. The first thing I could imagine was that the cancer is now in my spine.
>
> <u>Provider:</u> (**Assessing**) Did you ever have back pain like that before? Did it feel the same?
>
> <u>Patient:</u> Once about 10 years ago, I was moving a couch with my son and I went into spasm in exactly the same place.
>
> <u>Provider:</u> We were both younger then. Did it go away or did you get medical attention?
>
> <u>Patient:</u> It took 6 days to get better but on the third day, I panicked, and my family doctor got x-rays, which were fine. Dr. Jones thought it was a pulled muscle.
>
> <u>Provider:</u> (*Does a physical exam, including a thorough check of motor strength in both legs, looking for uneven weakness, rectal tone, and sensory changes in the legs.*) How are your bowel movements and urination?
>
> <u>Patient:</u> I still have the usual diarrhea. Urinating is still slow, but it is happening.
>
> <u>Provider:</u> (**Conveying**) Ten years ago, you didn't have prostate cancer, so it wasn't so scary. It's possible—even likely—that it is a pulled muscle now too. You don't

have any weakness or any changes in sensation that I can find. Are you comfortable if we wait a few more days to see if it gets better, stays the same, or gets worse? If it doesn't, we'll get a bone scan and an MRI, and check some fancy blood work. But for now, I think we should wait just a bit.

Patient: If you think it's not urgent, then "yes."

Provider: (**Support**) Just about everyone getting treated for cancer has a scare like this sooner or later, when something happens and immediately, we think the cancer has spread. Let's see how the next few days go before we do more tests.

When revealing a confirmed diagnosis, the SPIKES system is the best to use in its entirety.

▦ INTRODUCING THE ROLE OF CLINICAL TRIALS

Using the same prompts (**a**ssess, **c**onvey, **s**upport), the discussion of clinical trials is almost always uncomfortable. It takes more time than making a usual joint clinical decision. Patients can easily jump to a number of false conclusions. "He doesn't know what to do, so he's thinking about an experimental treatment." "I must be so bad off that she thinks there is no usual option left." "I am not a guinea pig." These are common responses, thought to oneself or actually said.

Provider (**Assess**): We've been struggling to slow down the growth of the spots in your lung. Each time we changed chemotherapy drugs, we've been able to hold it back only a little. At our research conference last week, I heard of a new combination of chemotherapies, one of which you haven't yet used. Would you consider making a change?

Patient (52-year-old woman with breast cancer and lung metastases): Will it help?

Provider: I'd like to think "yes," but I am not sure. The drug is a part of a new class of chemotherapies, but it is FDA approved only for cancer that starts in the lung. Because its effectiveness on breast cancer in the lung is not yet known, it is only given in a clinical trial. What do you know about clinical trials?

Patient: Is that the same as a research study? Are you thinking about this because there is no hope for me, doctor?

Provider: Not at all. I believe we both want to shrink those tumors as much as possible, even stop them from growing completely if possible. Have you reconsidered our original plan to treat the cancer with chemotherapy?

Patient: No, not yet. I am frustrated that the tumors are still there, but I am glad they didn't get me yet. I'd like to hear more.

Provider: (**Convey**) The new drug is called *dostopinib*. It works by slowing down or stopping the cells from growing by attacking certain receptors on the outside of the cell. Some women have gotten very good results, slowed their tumors right down, but there of course are some potential side effects.

Patient: What are they?

Provider: Most often a skin reaction, something like the pimples you had when you were a teenager, but there could be more of them and in more places. They can usually be controlled with some of the same things we use for acne, lotions, anti-inflammatories, and antibiotics. There will also be some extra visits and a bunch of questionnaires, but the extra attention from our research nurse can make up for your effort, at least in part. The extra medication will be paid for by the sponsor of the study, and they will even reimburse you for the travel costs for the extra visits.

Patient: If your wife or sister had to decide, how would you advise her?

Provider: (**Support**) I'd say that this is a good idea. If it seems too hard, you can pull out of the study at any time, and we'll go back to your regular chemotherapy, though it is best to try to finish the six rounds. We've been through a lot so far, and I believe that if this doesn't work, we still will have more to choose from in the future. This is not the last thing for you to try.

STARTING AND STOPPING EACH TREATMENT MODALITY

Changing from chemotherapy to RT seems like it would not be difficult, but it is actually one that sometimes causes significant distress. It is speculated that the change in routine is upsetting. It's comforting to know where to go, who the staff members are, and that they know you. The newness can be decreased if a patient knows where to park or get off the bus if it is in a different building and where the bathrooms are located. Not having the same intensity of contact with the current staff is also a little scary to some folks.

Provider: (**Assess and Convey**) After a week off, in 2 weeks, you'll be starting your radiation therapy. Some of my patients get a little frightened when they have to go to a new place. It is kind of expected. When you saw Dr. Smith for the consultation visit, did she show you around the treatment area?

Patient: Actually yes, her nurse did. They even showed me where to hang my clothes and get a gown. It's awfully cold down there!

Provider: (**Support**) The machines need to be cool. Bring a sweater and put it over your gown until you are called. Within time, they will get to know you, and you will feel at ease with the staff as you do with the chemo nurses.

PARADOXICAL DISTRESS AT THE END OF TREATMENT

Provider (radiation oncologist): (**Assess and Convey**) You've spent a long time down here with us in the last 6 weeks, coming five times a week. Will you be glad to stop coming so often?

Patient: Well, yes and no. I can't wait to my skin to stop being so raw, but there's something comforting about being here so often, having you check me and my progress every day. Almost like if something is going wrong, you'd know it right away. I'll miss that and feeling that I'm being active in fighting my cancer.

Provider: (**Support**) Many of our patients find they miss us the week after they stop the treatment, and they miss being checked so often. It's to be expected. We'll call you at home next week just to check in, and we'll see you the week after for follow-up. The radiation helps you long after you come in for treatment.

The Language of Failure

Virtually all of us have said it at one point or another. We probably heard it first in rounds as medical or nursing students. It started out innocently. "The surgery failed when the bleeding couldn't be stopped." "Emergency dialysis failed to restart the kidneys." "The atrioventricular (AV) shunt failed and dialysis had to be stopped." "He has end-stage liver failure."

These sound like reasonable ways to present findings. But somewhere, it got personalized. "The Taxol® failed to stop the ovarian cancer" became "She failed to get a response from the Taxol," and then, "She failed Taxol." Diagramming sentences goes in and out of favor, but having the verb *failed* right after the subject "she" erroneously can lead a patient to believe that it was somehow her fault, a weakness of the patient's moral character or fortitude.[30] What we say to each other (quietly) at the nurses' station or on the telephone can too easily become public when our cell call comes in the hospital elevator, in hallway discussions, or on bedside teaching rounds. Patients and caregivers alike who have not been inoculated in work rounds to the idiosyncratic use of the word are often offended and feel victimized. Caution is imperative with this quirk of language.

▩ THE THREE HARDEST PARTS OF YOUR DAY

Two of the three hardest communications often involve having to confirm a relapse, a recurrence, or a disease progression despite active treatment. It makes us all uncomfortable in some way. Colleagues have candidly discussed feeling like they have failed as healers, or that their specialty choice should have been one with more positive outcomes. Those very personal feelings are often clouded by fears that a patient (or well-meaning family member, usually from far away) will be quite angry. Such discussions are time consuming when we are ever more pressed for time, make it hard to plan in advance and then throw off an office schedule, or keep us at the hospital when we are late for office hours and the waiting room is backing up. Frequently, these discussions are followed by phone calls from questioning relatives, both those who are authorized via the Health Insurance Portability and Accountability Act (HIPAA) consent as well as those who are not. There may even be fear or threats of litigation stemming from the anger and disappointment.

The idea that effective communication skills are learned parallels the idea that we need to try to do things as well as we can even if we cannot change the outcome. In health care, doing the right thing as well as possible is often the secondary goal behind saving a life or helping to heal. In situations where cure or control of cancer is not possible, going about it the best way possible becomes the primary focus—"best way" for the patient and family as well as for the way we practice.

Revealing a Recurrence or Relapse

Knowing how disappointed patients, families, and providers are when disease has progressed despite everyone's best efforts, providers take the lead to focus on what can be done next. That sets a certain tone of cautious optimism, reaching to second- or third-line chemotherapies or some added radiation from a different approach. Surgical oncologists have recently been able to step in with ever more sophisticated techniques for metastasectomy in the lungs, liver, or brain. Interventional radiology and nuclear medicine in some settings can also offer competing treatments with CT-guided embolization or radioactive isotopes given systemically.

For providers, maintaining enthusiasm and personally feeling disappointed at the same time is a hard balancing act. On one hand, the public perception is the hope we "don't give up." On the other, all of us as providers, patients ourselves at times, hope that the offer for future intervention has real promise of helping. That equilibrium is hard to reach. Our challenge becomes to accurately characterize how effective any proposed treatment can be while not raising hopes excessively, which would result in everyone becoming frustrated again if the treatment underperforms.

Aligning and managing our expectations and those of the patient and family are a strategic challenge. We want to make sure that patients get every possible chance for the longest survival possible. Patients and families may be at odds with that goal for a variety of reasons. Perhaps they are suffering more than they admit. If the proper socially correct and expedient answer to "How are you?" is the automatic "Fine," then the level of specificity and degree of candor may not be accurate. Understandably, patients often do not want to let us down just as we don't want to let them down. Such courtesies can interfere with solid treatment planning.

Making a good treatment decision at the time of relapse or recurrence is a time when the forethought and discussion of having completed *What Is Important to Me* can be very helpful. One of the principles of advance care planning is that the individual who does so can change his or her mind at any point in the future. The degree to which our advance decisions are consistent over time is hard to track and study in oncology. Ditto and colleagues[31] interviewed older adults and then followed up with the same individuals 1 and 2 years later, finding that their preferences remained moderately stable over time. It can be argued that the immediacy of progressive disease during a life-threatening illness could encourage a change of preference, just as pregnant women who want analgesic-free deliveries ask for pain relief when the pain becomes severe during delivery.

The
LEARN
System©

p. 133
What Is
Important
To Me

Having *What Is Important to Me* as a basis for decision making helps as a starting point. *It is much easier than opening the conversation for the first time at such a critical moment. "Since the discussions you had with your family when you completed What Is Important to Me, have you had further thoughts about what you would want to do now?"* or a similar question elicits the stability of the prior-stated preferences.

When advance directives first came into use in the United States, there was a great resistance to having patient discussions and using them for the reasons still very much evident today: fear of patients losing hope and giving up prematurely, time invested to have the discussions, potential anger from patient and family, fear of litigation, and feelings of professional failure. It was common to see patients with whom a discussion of goals and values was very much necessary but not done because they were being offered the least toxic chemotherapy alternative or an extra dose of *spot radiation*, and discussion and planning was postponed. That approach seems to defer patient and family anger and disappointment, not avoid it.

Office Visits Can Recalibrate the Discussion

When the news is either good or bad, rather than rediscuss only at the junctures where tensions are high and big decisions need to be made, having *What Is Important to Me* discussed from the start, the easiest approach is to refer to the discussion regularly, not necessarily at every visit, but at most of them. "The goals of your treatment that we discussed before . . . any change?" or something like that in your own words makes it routine and so much easier when big decisions need to be made. Using *My Weekly Planner*, the trajectory of the effects of cancer and coping with it are evident in a glance, with the preparation done *before* the office visit.

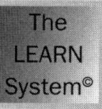

p. 141
My Weekly
Recovery
Planner

When Disease Control Is Not Possible

If assessing goals of care and planning is difficult at the time of recurrence or relapse, that difficulty is many times more challenging when patients' treatment is clearly not working. Sometimes, the toxicities are so profound that patients are "too sick to come in" or have an emergency hospital admission. At times, a patient or a family member may say so directly during their visit. Other times, which should be less prevalent with all of the preparatory work suggested, a family member will call you out of the room or pantomime behind the patient outside of his or her visual field to step outside or say silently, with accompanying hand signals of a major league baseball referee, "no more."

Your personal philosophy kicks in here in a very obvious way. If your personal sense of "Don't give up on me" means fourth- or fifth-line treatment, then the patient's preferences may not align with yours. In theory, the patient's preferences trump yours. In practice, and often without full discussion, recommendations for continued treatment with less effective strategies will follow. If your personal sense of "Don't give up on me" means "At this point, we will focus all of the efforts on making your quality of life as good as it can be," you may recommend that you continue to see the patient and have optimal symptom management as the main goal. You will know how to gauge the patient because you have gotten to know him or her from the start of care. Without the initial discussions starting at the first consult visit, such a discussion starting now will likely debase the patient and family and be very hard for you.

If you and your team are comfortable managing symptoms thoroughly, you would of course continue to do so. If you are not, there is help. Broaden your understanding of the concept and services of palliative care specialists; hospice and palliative care specialists are not just only effective for the last hours or days of life. At this point in care, you and your patient/family can benefit greatly from these experts' experience. Even suggesting a consult from a palliative care specialist requires a bit of patient and family education. That explanation should include that you would like a specialist consultation from the palliative care provider (the "symptom management expert"), and that does *not* mean you feel that death is imminent or close. Also, an assurance that you remain involved, coordinating care as you would with any other specialist, bypasses the idea that you are leaving the patient and family adrift. That is a great comfort because they have gotten to know and trust you (and you may even have looked forward to your encounters with them). Just as you took second seat when the patient's main treatment was with one of the other subspecialists, you can with the palliative care provider who will work with you and the larger team of providers. Good communication back and forth makes it possible, and the forms that you have used thus far (*What Is Important to Me, Communicator Sheets, Personal Health Records*) continue to be helpful.

If the managed care carrier will not authorize visits to both the palliative care specialist and you, keep in touch in some way such as a phone call from your office (the physician and nursing contact is optimal; nonclinical staff can also be a good link but cannot provide the medical guidance). If the patient is in the hospital but not on your service, a quick "Hello" and a "How are you doing?" means more than you can estimate.

The key point in this transition is that you and the team (including the palliative care provider) are *now going to put your full efforts into symptom management*. Stress what is being done, not what is being stopped. Using the term "keeping you comfortable" if the patient is still getting out of bed at home or participating in even limited activities could erroneously imply that death is approaching. So if possible, avoid those words until you believe a patient is closer to dying.

If you are unsure how to find a palliative care expert in your community, resources exist. Call or ask your staff to call over to the local hospice and see whom they recommend. Sometimes, it is the hospice medical director who also sees patients for symptom management outside of the hospice setting. Identify local practitioners who are board certified in hospice and palliative medicine (http://www.aahpm.org). In the newly revised 2012 standards for accreditation by the American College of Surgeons Commission on Cancer, a mechanism to triage and provide palliative care input is expected to be made mandatory over the next few years, so the staff at your accredited cancer center will know to whom they turn.

Patient Deaths

Author's Note: *If you've been in practice for a while, the skills of good communication around a patient's death may have become second nature and/or remain a distasteful part*

The LEARN System©

p. 143–150
My Recovery Plan Communicator

The LEARN System©

p. 168
Your Personal Health Record

of oncology practice. If like most of us these encounters leave us wanting, or when you have the opportunity to in-service new staff, the principles of good communication summarized are constant. This section may not be new to you but can be handy for teaching purposes as well as recalibrate your own skills. With new house staff beginning right before many more senior clinicians fire up their grills for the Fourth of July holiday, this primer may be a helpful teaching tool. It is not meant to undermine years of experience or your best practices!

This is the third hard part of a cancer provider's "day." It is, unfortunately, a basic task. All of us have been in this situation. For many providers, as we get more experienced and further along in practice, we sometimes get further away from the hardest tasks such as informing families of a patient death. With the current trend that has so limited hospital admission to the acutely sick and the uptick in referrals to hospice programs, *families are often calling us* to notify us a patient has died. Families are less trained for this charge than we are. This is one of the hardest things providers must master, and it often does not leave us feeling accomplished. But it *is a learned skill using the same principles being addressed in this text.* Today's medical care has us involved in three common circumstances in which we communicate about a patient's death: providers are the informant when a patient dies in the hospital; a family calls us to notify us; and/or another provider tells us, sometimes from the hospice, and we plan a follow-up call to the family.

Making the Call

In the inpatient teaching hospital setting, a member of the house staff calls us because we are rarely *in attendance* at the actual moment of death. Treatment bureaucracy sometimes detours the process of calling the attending physician of record. With the limitations on house staff hours, the medical student, intern, or resident whom you asked to call you has signed off once or twice, and in the triage of sign outs, the note to call you may not have been as important as the gastrointestinal (GI) bleed down the hall with hemoglobin of 5 gm/dl. And besides, by proxy, the trainee feels like (s)he failed, too, and puts the call low on the priority list of scut work. Depending on local laws and customs, during the interval between the death and the call to you, the nursing shift supervisor may have already notified the organ donor network that may have already been in touch with the family. If communication is effective and you are the first to call, follow the same principles: assess, convey, and support.

Provider: Hello Mrs. Jones, it's Dr. Smith. A lot has happened since we spoke a few hours ago, and I know it's late. Even more has happened since we saw each other in your husband's hospital room. (**Assess**) Has anyone called you in the last few hours?

Patient's wife: No, not since I left about 3 hours ago. It was 1:00 AM and I was okay to drive home but fell right asleep since I have been so overtired.

Provider: When I left, Mr. Jones was about the same, but after that, (**Convey**) he began to respond less to the staff, and his blood pressure dropped. Based upon what he told us when he could make his wishes known, he did not want to be moved to the intensive care unit if the interventions there would make him sicker and not better. The ICU fellow did stop by and confirmed with the senior resident who called me and the nurse to say that we would maintain his fluids and give medicine to ease the shortness of breath. This worked for a little while, but despite everyone's best efforts, his breathing could not keep up and he died. The staff there assures me he was comfortable.

(**Support**) Sometimes, news like this is better face-to-face, but because of the late hour, we didn't want you to come back when you were so overtired, and the nurse confirmed you had suspected he may not last the night and had private time with him before you left. We've been through a lot these moments during the last few years since George's lung cancer was diagnosed, and you've been able to be by his side all the way through when he was more aware of how you stayed by him. (*Pause*)

Patient's wife: Yes, it's been a long haul. Thank you for all you've done for our family, Dr. Smith. I will call the nurse now and will wait at least 'till 5:00 to call my kids. They all visited today, too, and we went to the funeral home yesterday.

Provider: I am so sorry for your loss. This is one of those moments in life that you'll remember for some time. I will tell the office staff in the morning. Can you or one of your children call with the funeral arrangements when they are confirmed? Thank you so much, and I can speak for the whole staff that we are sorry for your family's loss. Get some rest after you speak with the nurse. Good night.

Another idealized interchange but it illustrates good communication. Although the provider spoke a lot more, he gave time for response and for listening. In our haste, especially when we are less experienced, we may only talk or move through the conversation as if it were a court hearing. In this example, Dr. Smith does not just give the bad news quickly but goes through the steps and the processes. It is a similar interchange if an emergency room staffer calls a relative after an unexpected accident, and the relative lives too far away to come in. (Otherwise, it's something like, "This is Dr. Intern at local hospital. We haven't met, but I need to let you know that Mrs. Doe has been injured in a car accident. She's lost a lot of blood and is getting transfused and then some x-rays. Best if you come here as soon as you can and ask for the emergency department. We're doing everything possible now.")

When the phone call is completed, save 30 seconds to stop what you're doing (hopefully, you were not speaking on your headset while you were driving). Be still for a few seconds—30 seconds or so. Realize how pivotal your call has been in this family's life, and how each patient touches you, some more than others. Such a pause allows us to continue to the next patient and the next, exhaling a bit of CO_2 with a bit of respect for participating in the moment. We're not a Fortune 500 manufacturer, and we're not just shipping microchips. The human services we provide affect us and society in a much more personal way.

Confirming but Not the First Call

Similarly, with some minor changes if a resident calls first, you might say, "I understand that Dr. Resident just got off the phone with you. I can speak for my staff to say we are sorry for your family's loss. Are there any questions that Dr. Resident was unable to answer? You just met her a few hours ago. (*Pause*) Will you call the office . . ."

Family Calls You

Provider: Dr. Smith, yes Mrs. Jones. The receptionist tells me you were holding on the line. I was just finishing up with someone in the office, sorry for the delay. Has there been a change in Mr. Jones's condition at home? The hospice nurse called early this morning to report that he was comfortable but not responsive. (*Pause*)

Patient's wife: Yes, Dr. Smith, he died just a few minutes ago. The kids are here and some neighbors. The chaplain is on her way over. I have to call the funeral home so I can't linger, but I just wanted you to know.

Provider: We here are so sorry for your family's loss. Is there anything we can do for you right now? (*Pause*) You must be filled with emotions. These past few weeks have been hard on your family. When you have made the funeral arrangements, can someone call here and let us know what they are? We are so sorry for your loss.

Heard After the Fact From the Hospice Program or Another Facility Where Admitted

One of the oddities in the bureaucracy that plagues hospice programs is that the program's attending of record must be notified of a patient's death, and the social worker and chaplain are dispatched to the home or call there. Often, the referring doctor is *not* the attending of record because (s)he does not attend the every 2-week interdisciplinary team discussions and sign the multitude of forms to conform to federal regulations put into place when Medicare developed home hospice. As more record keeping is electronic, providers who are not on the hospice staff do not have access to the electronic record, so the staff providers must keep up with the paperwork, taking the referring or community provider out of the loop for a call. Most programs have a manual override and a way to clearly indicate in the record, on paper or electronically, to call the referring or community provider to alert him or her of the death. When you make the referral, make clear if/how/when you want to be notified. Keep in mind that instant messaging and short social media such as Twitter do not have the highest level of privacy yet, and most likely, are not acceptable. Notification of such information through the social media also loses the personal touch that is so vital at that moment and the gravitas of the event.

Your call to the family remains a variant of the inpatient call.

(**Assess**): Mrs. Jones, it's Dr. Smith. I understand my office got a call from nurse X, chaplain Y, or social worker Z yesterday that Mr. Jones died/passed on/ (_____; *phrase you believe fits best*). (**Convey**) I can speak for the staff when I say we are sorry for your loss. (*Pause*) (**Support**) These are not easy times. Is there anything I or the office staff can help you with right now?

Use the 30-second pause and take a deep breath after these calls, too. (It really works!) You will be able to move to the next task a little more easily. Become familiar with the local procedures of the organ donor network. House staff and hospital nursing staff in most locales no longer discuss organ donation or harvest because it is perceived as a conflict of interest when caring for someone to help them live. Also, be aware of the local health codes that probably dictate how long a patient may stay in the hospital unit after death and if there is any flexibility in your hospital. There is often reasonable accommodation for particular religious practices of the prevailing groups in your community, and it helps to be familiar with them ahead of time.

Similarly, a call from another facility to which the patient was admitted under someone else's care can spur a similar interchange.

Communication Further After a Death

Speak with your staff to see what is most comfortable. Oncology specialists often cannot attend every funeral of patients who have died. Some prefer to do so. There are a few models, and these vary from a rural setting to the exurbs to the suburbs and the inner city. Some groups attend on a rotating basis. Some practices send a personalized form or handwritten note; others have preprinted cards. There is a natural tension in attending funerals.[32] It is almost impossible to go to all of them. How do you decide? Is there an element of favoritism in such decisions? Is it basic courtesy where you practice? What do you say? Will attendees blame you for not controlling the cancer or thank you for your efforts? If staff members go to funerals, who is covering the chemotherapy suite or radiation center? Is staffing adequate for time away for funerals? Lots of questions and practice variations.

Especially outside of dense urban areas, you will run into a deceased patient's relatives when you least expect it in the supermarket or at the gym. Use the same principles: assess, convey, and support. Your script is not prewritten, but your approach is learned, just like doing a history and physical.

▪ *READ THIS*: REALLY UNDERSTANDING HOSPICE

The obstacles that discourage referral to hospice programs are the same as those involved in a referral to a palliative care consult. Feeling like a professional failure; myths and misunderstandings about hospice care; fear of angering patients, families, and caregivers; fear of litigation; and the perception of "giving up" all work together to everyone's detriment.

The myths about hospice care abound. They include "Hospice is a place to go to die—and they are not very nice places," "A patient must be DNR (do not resuscitate)," "A patient must die within 6 months," "Hospice does nothing but give morphine," "Hospice care does not allow for admission if necessary," "I can't remain in charge of the care once the patient elects hospice," and "I can no longer get paid for the care I give." These ideas are *untrue*; they are *myths*.

When hospice care became an entitlement under Medicare, public policy makers, many Medicaid, and private insurance programs sought to *demedicalize* end-of-life care, taking it out of the inpatient setting that is best to diagnose and treat illnesses. The inpatient mandate to figure out what is wrong with a patient using active diagnostic testing and move patients through the system and home as quickly as possible is antithetical to good end-of-life care. Based on the system honed in the United Kingdom, hospice became a home-based program with continuity of care on an inpatient unit, respite unit, in a skilled nursing facility, or at a homelike residence. Its main goal is comfort care for the patient and family/caregivers, with a large effort to coordinate care and provide the services thought to be optimal at the end of life. It brought services *to the patient and family*, avoiding travel to separate providers or facilities.

Nursing care and coordination is front and center, with psychosocial support provided by counselors of a variety of disciplines including pastoral care, volunteer services, and all medications and durable and disposable medical equipment necessary to treat the illness that is the most likely to lead to death. A limited number of home health/hospice aide services are provided for the patient and as respite for caregivers. Prescription drugs, supplies, and equipment are delivered to the home; no need to go pick them up. Paradoxically, patients are free to travel (in contrast to when they access the standard home care benefit, which limits them to being homebound except for doctor visits to qualify). For a short visit, through a courteous and cooperative system, the local hospice will supply services with advance warning. For longer stays, care is transferred.

Physician services can remain with the referring provider of any specialty or assumed by the hospice medical director. Consultations are provided as necessary for the ongoing plan of care that is reviewed at least once every 14 days by the hospice team.

Patients do agree to surrender their usual medical coverage of treatment *only for the illness that is likely to cause death, not for all of their benefits.* That management is now assumed by the hospice team, under your orders if you stay in charge or a Hospice Medical Director. There have been few co-pays until recently, and those remain minimal. In the words of Carolyn Cassin, the executive director of the National Hospice Working Group, "This is the richest benefit of any managed care contract known." As in a managed care system, admission to the hospital related to the hospice benefit must be authorized by the program at their contracted facility.

So why is this benefit accessed too late or not at all? No definitive study corroborates that the myths are the backbone of the resistance. It's not a perfect system. Upon referral, the referring provider (still a physician under the federal guidelines, even though hospice is a nursing-focused entity) must believe and sign documentation that (s)he believes that the patient will die within 6 months *if the disease runs its usual course.* That is misunderstood to mean that we have the ability to predict with great certainty who will die and who won't and when. Under Medicare guidelines, a patient with an illness who is likely to die within 6 months if the disease runs its usual course, there are two 90-day periods of benefit approval, *plus an unlimited* number of 60-day periods providing that the illness is still present *and there has been functional decline.*

When a patient is on hospice care, you will receive frequent calls from the nurse coordinator for orders. That is true, but you can (and should be) seeing the patient in your office or at home. You bill for those visits, *and with the right modifier suffix for the current procedural therapy (CPT) code for the visit, the bill gets routed the right way by your local Medicare fiscal intermediary and you are paid.* Whether you do house calls or not, your continuity with the patient and family is essential and becomes a chance to engage in what may now be considered hands-on, "old-fashioned" doctoring and nursing without a computer screen between you and your patient.

Rest assured that no one from a local authority to the Centers for Medicare and Medicaid Services will call or e-mail to complain that your predictive abilities need a tune-up or your patient lived too long. Patients do sometimes get better despite having a life-threatening diagnosis and at times do not show enough *decline* to stay on the program. As seemingly ridiculous as that has become, you may hear that your patient is "not sick enough" and sometimes that is simply a case of more crisp documentation (appended photos are acceptable even in an electronic medical record). At times, patients will go back to their regular insurance and then reenroll when they show decline. Sometimes, patients and families feel they are being abandoned at a time that they are so sick, so the documentation needs to be as full and complete as possible to support ongoing hospice care.

Disappointment from the patient and family side often grows from the shared sense of failure or guilt that they are "giving up." That disappointment often is misplaced in the misunderstanding that the program does not send a nurse or home care/hospice aide to provide care 24 hours a day, 7 days a week. The services are linked to medical necessity and reducing caregiver burnout, often about 20 hours a week, until the last days of life, when the home care can be boosted to 24-hour coverage if needed. In some ways, that creates an unexpected opportunity for some degree of closeness between the patient and family at a time that cannot be recaptured, but *is a burden* on working families who are multitasking. Most families rise to the occasion, making patchwork schedules and calling in favors from extended family, friends, and community members.

▦ FINDING OUT ABOUT WHAT SERVICES ARE AVAILABLE IN YOUR AREA

Because Certificates of Need in most states are given to a certain number of hospice programs in a given county, it is highly likely that you have one or a variety of programs to choose for referrals. Ask the medical director or director of patient care services to make a (brief) presentation at an office meeting or at a time when the schedule is thinner. Your patients and families will let you know which services were good and which were under par. As with any extended care program or facility, maintaining referrals keeps the programs afloat, encouraging outreach. Also ask about the availability of a palliative care expert close to your practice.

▦ MAKING THE REFERRAL

Although patients and families can self-refer to hospice programs, part of the referral process involves your certification that the patient has a life expectancy of 6 months or less *if the disease runs its usual course*. The noncancer criteria are somewhat more nebulous, but the cancer criteria are relatively straightforward. How the idea is introduced is harder.

▦ ELIGIBILITY CRITERIA FOR PATIENTS WITH CANCER

Hospice eligibility for patients with cancer includes patients who have metastatic disease, a decline in performance status, and who are no longer receiving treatment that will extend life expectancy or who have declined cancer treatment. For patients with hematological cancers, testing has shown an equivalent decline in marrow function or relapse. Often, there is unintentional weight loss at the same time.

■ HAVING "THE DISCUSSION"

The approach can most easily be followed using the *ACS* steps: assess, convey, and support.

Provider: (**Assess**) We have gone through a number of treatments (specify) and we are at an important decision point. From what I have seen, the last treatment(s) have given you side effects without much control over the cancer. Is that your sense, too?

Patient: Well, yes, but I am scared to stop fighting the cancer. You're not just going to give up on me, are you?

Provider: We want to do things that make you feel better, not worse. Have you considered changing the focus of our care so that we devote our full attention to treating your symptoms so you can function as well and as fully as possible?

Patient: I've been thinking the same thing but was scared to ask you. What were you thinking?

Provider: (**Convey**) Your insurance coverage includes some home care benefits that will bring the services you need to your home, including specialty level care, equipment, medications, and even some practical help. Many people don't understand that these added services are part of your hospice benefit. Many people think that hospices are a place to go or that they help out in the last days or hours of life, so they are scared by even the mention of the word. Hospice care can continue for a long time if it is helpful. We're not giving up on caring for you, but all of us want you to get the care you need at this point in your cancer treatment.

(**Support**) It may be a surprise that we are discussing this option now. Most patients are disappointed when we need to have this discussion. Can you explain this to your family (those not there) members who have not come with you today, and we can continue the discussion in person or by telephone? In the meantime, can I ask someone from the hospice program to get some information to you?

Of course, this is an idealized interchange, but the gist of the encounter is universally germane. Focused listening techniques may be helpful here, asking the patient or a family member to repeat what he or she has just heard. Often, when we are upset and in emotional situations, we don't take in all the information. This is one instance where you want to be certain that the listener has an accurate and clear understanding of what you have said.

Patients and family members may cry, be angry, or relieved. Using the information in *What Is Important to Me*, you can gauge their response. We have all seen this transition handled less than optimally in the past, and that includes statements like "There is nothing more to offer" and "Go get your affairs in order." You will develop your own version of this discussion.

Section III

Working With Your Patients

Tools for Survivorship

My Recovery Plan helps patients and families anticipate what they need to consider, discuss *in advance*, and organize valuable personal information necessary to make optimal choices during the work-up, treatment and beyond.

The LEARN System focuses on information that patients and families can and need to learn during treatment from their providers about their particular clinical course, with an emphasis on five basic tasks:

L – focus regularly on an aspect of **l**iving outside of the time spent in treatment for perspective

E – **e**ducation; learning as much as fits your style about your cancer, and what you can do to recover from treatment

A – physical **a**ctivity to the extent able during and after treatment minimizes deconditioning afterwards

R – using periods of **r**est and energy conservation to optimize energy during and after treatment

N – good **n**utrition pared with the limitations of treatment to maintain energy and healing.

The LEARN System organizes what we often ask patients to do in a more formal way, and provides some tools for patients and families to do so.

Components of The LEARN System
L Living
E Education
A Activity
R Rest
N Nutrition

▓ FORMS THAT EXPEDITE THOUGHT AND DISCUSSION: GOAL SETTING *EARLY* AT THE START OF CARE

Quickly familiarize yourself with the forms that patients and their families may be using as prompts for questions. The forms are reproduced at the back of this book to be copied and used in your office. They are also included in *LEARN to Live Through Cancer: What You Need to Know and Do* written expressly for patients and families.

▦ FORMS TO BE COMPLETED BEFORE THE INITIAL CONSULTATION

WHAT IS IMPORTANT TO ME

I believe that life is precious and I want to continue living as well as I can for as long as I can.

At the time of my cancer diagnosis, I want to go through all of the necessary consultations and tests to determine, with the best medical expertise and judgment available:

- ■ The kind of cancer I have: _____
- ■ Where it is:
  - ❑ Locally advanced (where it started)
  - ❑ Lymph nodes
  - ❑ Other body systems; locations: _____
  _____

With treatment, it is my understanding that:

- ❑ I can be cancer-free for five years or more.
- ❑ I will likely need to be more treatment within the next five years.
- ❑ I will be on maintenance treatment for the rest of my life.

CHOOSE ONE (1) OF THE FOLLOWING:

- ❑ I am willing to do anything and everything necessary to control my cancer.

- ❑ I am interested in preserving my quality of life as well as surviving my cancer. With each proposed change in my treatment plan, please save a few minutes so we can discuss the benefit of the treatment and how I can expect to feel.

- ❑ I am more interested in preserving my quality of life if it is unlikely for me to survive my cancer for more than:

  ❑ 3 months   ❑ 6 months   ❑ 1 year   ❑ 2 years

Know:

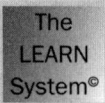

The LEARN System©

p. 133
What Is
Important
To Me

What Is Important to Me helps patients and families have hard, personal discussions outside of your office so that you can review their preferences, rather than have the complete discussion in your consult room. It helps define approach and values, not individual treatment decisions. More complete information is found in Chapter 6.

Do:

When submitted with documents and records prior to your appointment with family input or privately, you and your staff can review it in advance, using face-to-face time at the initial appointment to clarify the responses.

FAMILY HISTORY FORM

Patient Name: _____ D.O.B. _____ Today's Date: _____

Directions: Please list **all** of your <u>biological</u> (blood) relatives **below including those who have not had cancer**. **If someone is deceased, please put an asterisk** (*) in the age column next to the age at death. Use an additional page if you need extra space. You may not know each piece of information we are asking for. If you are unsure of something, give your best guess and put a question mark (?) next to it. It may be helpful to contact family members who may know additional information, but if this is not possible, we will do our best with the information you can give us.

Relationship to You	Name or initials	Current age or age at death (mark* if deceased)	Date of birth (approximate if unsure)	Cancer type (s) If person has not had cancer, leave blank.	Age at cancer diagnosis
Your Children	List your children below. In the first column, circle son or daughter for each child.				
Son / Daughter					
Son / Daughter					
Son / Daughter					
Son / Daughter					
Son / Daughter					
Son / Daughter					
Your Brothers and Sisters	List each of your brothers and sisters below. If half-sibling, specify which parent you share.				
Brother / Sister					
Brother / Sister					
Brother / Sister					

Know:

The **Family History** can be completed before a patient's initial consult if your office provides it in advance of the appointment on paper or electronically. Many patients need to poll family members to see what Uncle Johnny had as they themselves do not know. Because cancer as an entity was not addressed in some cultures openly, asking a family to quiz relatives at the start of care standardizes the process.

Do:

Much of the information that you need to decide if a referral for screening by a genetic counselor, whether or not actual genetic testing is indicated is now part of your record. Even if the referral is made when treatment is over, you have the historical information for consideration at the proper time.

The
LEARN
System©

p. 135–137
Family
History
Form

IMPORTANT REVELATIONS TO MY TREATMENT TEAM

Please complete as many of the items that pertain to you and your family. Some of this information may be personal or embarrassing. Being candid will ease your treatment so that your needs can be best anticipated.

PART 1

Personal information:

I am the kind of person who likes *a lot/little* information.

Family history of important conditions that will affect my treatment:

     Cancer (type, age) (For more detailed family history, see Family History Form)

     Serious depression (even if never treated)

     Significant drinking or drug (substance abuse problems)

Conditions important to consider during cancer treatment (see worksheet):

     Motion sickness (trains, planes, car, bus)

     Comfort level in closed spaces

     Nausea/vomiting during pregnancy

Know:

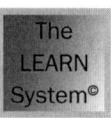

The
LEARN
System©

p. 138–139
Important
Revelations
To My
Treatment
Team

Important Revelations to My Treatment Team easily collects information that is sometimes omitted from an initial history because it may not seem pertinent at the moment. This form documents seemingly minor details that become important as treatment progresses.

Do:

Use this information to personalize care. A more accurate depiction of alcohol and tobacco use, as well as specifics about a history of motion sickness, will help drive some of the ancillary decisions that are made with a patient and family, such as how aggressively to prepare a patient with anti-emetics for the first round of chemotherapy, and a reinforce decision-making style that directs shared decision-making.

◼ ISSUES PATIENTS MAY BRING UP AT THE FIRST CONSULT

QUESTIONS I WANT ANSWERED

How will I feel?

Will I recover and be myself?

What will the treatment include?

Can I continue to work?

How can I arrange for a second opinion? (No offense, please, but this is serious and I need to know.)

Who can help with my kids? Will I need help at home?

What do I need to do during my treatment? Eating, exercise?

What will be affected by the cancer and by the treatments?

What about vitamins and supplements?

What are *clinical trials*?

What is important to me now?

What do I have to do to get better?

When will I feel OK again? Will I be the same?

Will the cancer come back?

Know:

Questions I Want Answered gives a voice to questions that patients and families ask routinely. It is by no means a full list. Each question does not pertain to every patient or at every stage of illness. They are included not to scare but to legitimize the concerns that patients and families have. Often, under the guise of "protecting" others, family members and patients alike do not want to mention various issues, as if it is not being thought about anyway. Many of us grew up with the children's story, *The Emperor's New Clothes,* a Hans Christian Anderson classic tale that condemns the person who voices the obvious. In the current climate where transparency in medical care can be at odds with protecting patients and families from undue suffering, the elements of *What Is Important to Me* and *Questions I Want Answered* may not be for everyone, but lend an experienced voice to those families who are ready.

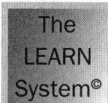

The LEARN System©

p. 140 Questions I Want Answered

Do:

No one has all of the answers, nor can all of the issues be discussed on the first visit or in any one visit. It will guide future discussions.

▣ AT THE START OF TREATMENT WITH ANY MODALITY:
SURGERY, CHEMOTHERAPY, RADIATION THERAPY
AND AT *REGULAR* INTERVALS
(DETERMINED BY TREATMENT REGIMEN)

MY WEEKLY RECOVERY PLANNER
Using The LEARN System®

Copy this form regularly to set your course and chart your progress.
Check which stage of recovery you are in:

☐ post-operative   ☐ right after treatment
　☐ chemotherapy ☐ radiation therapy   ☐ more than three months after treatment
　☐ combinations of above

Living	Do:	
	Done:	
Education	Do:	
	Done:	
Activity	Do:	
	Done:	
	Do:	

Know:

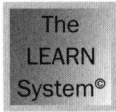

The
LEARN
System©

p. 141
My Weekly
Recovery
Planner

My Weekly Planner is a simple five-box form to help patients and families set goals for each week in each of the domains of The LEARN System. It can be reviewed at the end of each week to show progress, particularly in each of the areas, and can be used electronically or on paper. The overarching box for **L**iving raises it to a prominent position on the form and for life planning to include some activity that is meaningful or even enjoyable to balance the investment in cancer therapy.

Do:

More for the patient to track his or her goals for the week, it may or may not be shared at follow-up visits. Asking to see it reinforces your endorsement. Share this responsibility with your nurse, who has likely asked about these elements anyway.

DISTRESS THERMOMETER

Name:_____
Date: _____

Before you see your Nurse/Doctor, please complete this form. We would like to know how you are feeling and your concerns.

FIRST:
Please circle the number (0-10) that best describes *how much distress* you have been experiencing in the past week including today.

[name label]

```
10 ── Extreme distress
 9
 8
 7
 6
 5
 4
 3
 2
 1
 0 ── No distress
```

THEN: Please indicate WHICH of the following is a cause of distress. A staff member may call you to follow-up. At what telephone number would you like to be called?_____

Practical	**Physical**
☐ Housing	☐ Pain
☐ Insurance	☐ Nausea
☐ Work/school	☐ Fatigue [RN/MD: Hg:___ Hct:___]
☐ Transportation	☐ Sleep
☐ Child care	☐ Getting around
	☐ Bathing/dressing

Know:

The **Distress Thermometer** is adapted from the National Comprehensive Cancer Network's Distress Management Guidelines[33]. It is the prototype for an efficient tool that is both qualitative and quantitative. The global rating of 0–10 (0–3: mild; 4–6: moderate; ≥ 7: severe) may be for one or more of the items. It is designed as a triage tool, to help you and the clinical staff focus your time and attention.

Do:

Generally, patients and families take a few seconds to complete this form in the waiting room upon arrival. Placed on top of your chart (face down, of course for privacy) along with an Encounter Form for billing (if you use one), scan it quickly just as you are going to enter the exam room or infusion area. It gives you a general "heads-up" so you can direct your efforts without having to anticipate what to do. Other staff who may better address individual items (nursing, social work, office manager, nutritionist) can also be alerted to a specific need based upon the items endorsed.

The LEARN System©

p. 142
Distress
Thermometer

Know:

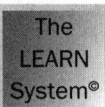

The **Journal** page is formatted for written expression or artistic endeavors. Its use encourages patients to record their reactions to their situation. Patients can use this to chart their course in words, doodles, or whatever medium they prefer.

Do:

The
LEARN
System©

p. 151
Journal
Page:
Charting My
Course

Nothing, as patients will likely keep this form private.

MY RECOVERY PLAN COMMUNICATOR
BREAST CANCER

Name: _____

Date: _____

Today and in the last three (3) days:

Energy: ☐ Good ☐ Fair ☐ Poor

Weight _____ ☐ Gain ☐ Loss   Appetite: ☐ Good ☐ Fair ☐ Poor

Hot Flashes ☐ Yes: ____ per day ☐ No

Chemo: Date last given: _____
White cell count _____ Hemoglobin _____ Platelet count _____
[ ] erythropoeitin   [ ] filgastrim
☐ Nausea or vomiting
☐ Pins and needles or numbness anywhere, place: _____

Radiation: Skin reaction ☐ yes ☐ no   [ ] Aquaphor® [ ] Aloe Vera

[ ] Biafene® [ ] Silvadene® [ ] Other: _____

Surgery: Postoperative healing ☐ good ☐ not healing

Medications: name and dose: _____

_____

_____

Know:

Communicator Sheets ease the burden of passing information back and forth to colleagues who do not share an electronic or paper medical record with your practice. Patients and families carry it between providers, saving staff time from scanning or faxing. Its use can avoid duplicative CBCs, other tests or delays. The sheets at the end of this book are tailored to the most common cancers. A general template is also included for less common scenarios.

Do:

Involve your nurse and use this form along with any discharge information from the infusion or radiation suite. For privacy, you may want to put the form in an envelope. Record the information brought to you from one of the other providers in your progress note, chemotherapy flow chart, or status check form during radiation therapy.

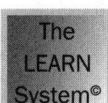

The LEARN System©

p. 143–150
My Recovery Plan Communicator

▦ WHEN TREATMENT FINISHES

PERSONAL HEALTH RECORD

Last Name: First Name:
DOB: Age: Gender: Date:
Day Phone: Evening Phone:
Address: City: State: Zip:
Email:
My Insurance: Policy #:

Spouse/Relative/Caretaker: Phone:
Health Care Proxy: Phone:

MEDICAL INFORMATION

Type of Cancer: Date of diagnosis:
Staging   T: N: M:

My Health Care Team   **Phone:**   **Email:**
Medical Oncologist:
Radiation Oncologist:
Surgeon:
Fellow:
Nurse Practitioner:
Integrative Oncology Nurse:
Speech/Swallowing Therapist:
Pain/Symptom Management:
Dentist/Orthodontist:
Nutritionist:
Physical Therapist:
Social Worker:

Treatments received:
Surgical Procedures:

Chemotherapy: ☐   (mg)   ☐   (mg)   ☐   (mg)
             ☐   (mg)   ☐   (mg)   ☐ other
Freq: Total Dose:

Radiation Therapy:
Area treated:
☐ External Beam Radiation Therapy
(EBRT)   Last Date: Dose:
☐ Brachytherapy   Last Date: Procedure: Dose:

FOLLOW-UP APPOINTMENTS:
Follow-ups: *Remember to follow up with your providers on a regular schedule*

☐ Surgical: ☐ Radiation Oncology: ☐ Medical Oncology:
☐ Cancer Supportive Services: ☐ Pain/Symptom Management: ☐ Nutrition:

☐ Speech/Swallowing Therapy: ☐ Physical Therapy: ☐ Social Work:

☐ Dental:

Know:

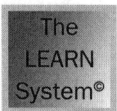

The LEARN System©

p. 168
Your
Personal
Health
Record

Personal Health Records (PHR)s or **survivorship care plans** are coming into regular use at cancer centers across the country to fulfill a clinical void and in response to the IOM Report. The PHR reinforces the patient's and family's responsibility in the recovery process, and advises them about local resources. PHRs are also reviewed in greater detail in the Communication chapter.

Do:

With your staff, have copies of the form ready for use in a vertical file, or scanned into your electronic medical record. When using paper forms, enlarge them in the copy machine to standard 8.5 x 11 size. develop a system to collect information for this form. To simplify the task, you will be including many of the same points in your Treatment Summary note for which it can serve as a template.

▦ WITH REFRACTORY OR PROGRESSIVE DISEASE

MY PERSONAL AFFAIRS

❑ Last will and testament

❑ Health care proxy, living will, or other advance medical directive acceptable in your state

❑ Power of attorney

❑ List of bank accounts, pensions, life insurance policies (with review of the beneficiaries or "in trust for..." designations)

❑ Special accommodations for dependent children or elderly

❑ Thoughts about memorial services, burial or cremation, including list of invitees

❑ Wording of obituary

❑ Letters, audio or video recordings you would like to leave for loved ones on upcoming milestones in their lives: school graduations, marriages, births, or other such momentous personal occasions

❑ "How I want you to remember me" thoughts. Written or recorded. This is something almost always neglected because the people who love you the most are afraid to bring it up to avoid scaring you that you are closer to death than you would believe (another conspiracy of silence thing)

❑ "What I know that you may not": genealogy, family history, stories, Grandma's cookie recipes; whatever is significant in your family's life

❑ "Permission slips": Regarding very personal and deep family issues: permission to move from the family house when the time is right; permission for a spouse to date or remarry (grist for many a made-for-television movie), permission to go back to school to finish a degree. There are many variations on this theme.

❑ Thank you's

Know:

My Personal Affairs puts in checklist format the tasks that must be accomplished when the old adage, "time to put your affairs in order" becomes necessary. This form is helpful for those patients whose cancer does not respond to treatment, despite everyone's best efforts progresses, the transition to focus primarily on symptom management and the involvement of hospice.

Do:

Personal form for patient and family informational purposes. Requires no action.

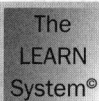

The
LEARN
System©

p. 203
My Personal
Affairs

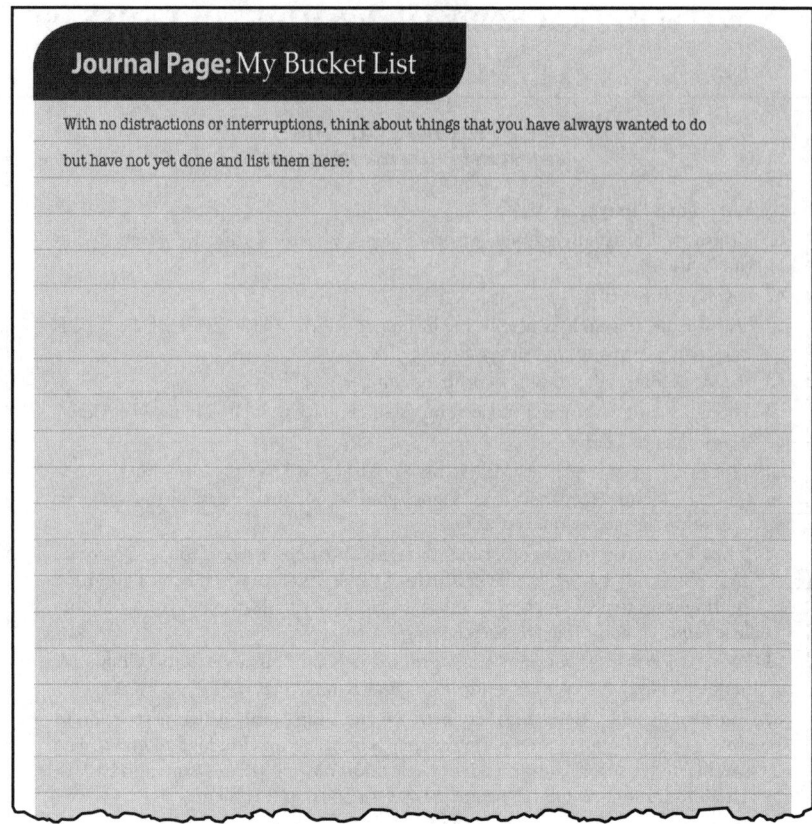

Know:

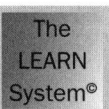

The **My Bucket List** form emanates from a rite of passage further acculturated by a recent comedic-drama film. The form encourages thought to plan memorable activities whose opportunities may sometime be past due.

Do:

p. 204
My Bucket
List

Personal form for patient and family informational purposes. Requires no action.

▓ AT VARYING POINTS IN TREATMENT

FIVE WISHES

T here are many things in life that are out of our hands. This Five Wishes document gives you a way to control something very important—how you are treated if you get seriously ill. It is an easy-to-complete form that lets you say exactly what you want. Once it is filled out and properly signed it is valid under the laws of most states.

What Is Five Wishes?

Five Wishes is the first living will that talks about your personal, emotional and spiritual needs as well as your medical wishes. It lets you choose the person you want to make health care decisions for you if you are not able to make them for yourself. Five Wishes lets you say exactly how you wish to be treated if you get seriously ill. It was written with the help of The American Bar Association's Commission on Law and Aging, and the nation's leading experts in end-of-life care. It's also easy to use. All you have to do is check a box, circle a direction, or write a few sentences.

How Five Wishes Can Help You And Your Family

- It lets you talk with your family, friends and doctor about how you want to be treated if you become seriously ill.

- Your family members will not have to guess what you want. It protects them if you become seriously ill, because they won't have to make hard choices without knowing your wishes.

- You can know what your mom, dad, spouse, or friend wants. You can be there for them when they need you most. You will understand what they really want.

Know:

Five Wishes is another useful tool for in end-of-life care planning. It includes information usually found on LivingWills or Health Care Proxies (Health Care Power of Attorney), and more specifics about personal choices about end-of-life care.

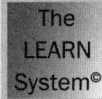

The LEARN System©

Do:

Use with or in place of forms in your locality. A list of states where the form is legally accepted is embedded into the form. Access to these forms off hours or for on-call staff is critical. Scan or file a copy where it is available outside of usual office hours. Scanning and depositing on a shared drive accessible from home or hospital is ideal.

p. 205
Five Wishes

The LEARN System Components: Finding Meaning and Purpose to Sustain Oneself During Treatment ("Living")

The LEARN acronym puts *Living* first, for it is the most elusive component of successful survivorship. Just as important documents have a preamble, books have an introduction, and health care institutions feature their mission statement front and center: *Living* is served best in the first position. *Living* may actually serve to crystallize the overarching themes in one's life that influence the choices we make for daily activities and outlook. One may wonder why a theme is necessary. Veteran survivors have affirmed that during the times they are most symptomatic from treatment, they find it helpful to have something on which to focus that reinforces the reasons to endure treatment. The thought processes and planning for the L component make up the information source to be tapped at the times when energy and motivation are insufficient to do so.

▩ THINK FOR THE LONG TERM

The theme of *Living* has two main purposes. *It asks a patient to clarify for himself or herself the elements of life that make the immediate investment in treatment worthwhile.* That is often not such an easy concept to discover or reveal. Rarely does one stop to do so in the midst of the busyness of daily life to take stock. Having such a rallying point becomes even more of a challenge once treatment starts, with many added activities that accompany each modality of treatment that may serve as distraction from our personal values.

Each patient may be able to set pen to paper and identify such life goals. Some may not. Some may—and should—instead open up the dialogue with close family and friends who may be able to size up the situation a bit more dispassionately and objectively. This type of discussion rarely happens. It also serves as a natural starting point to the domains brought up by *What Is Important to Me* focusing on what the next few weeks or months will be like if treatment is successful and effective, and beginning to think about end-of-life care if treatment is unsuccessful. *Living* self-assessment and discussions also serve as the compass for long-term survivorship, providing the first step to make longer term commitments to general health promotion through diet, exercise, smoking cessation, and alcohol minimization.

Patients sometimes are candid enough to describe their nighttime fears that plague them when they cannot fall asleep or stay asleep, fears that almost always seem more ominous and foreboding at night. Having the framework of *Living* gives a foundation to balance out such worry.

The LEARN System©

p. 133
What Is Important to Me

When cancer treatment delves into an existential area, traditionally, medical providers often take a deep breath and a step back. Clearly outside of our training, the fabric of one's life is traditionally material for the clergy or psychotherapist. No one is advocating that such discussions take up precious office time, with more than enough to cover during an ever decreasing time for the office visit. Advising, mentioning that it is helpful to have goals of living, not simply goals of care, is often enough to provide the impetus for patients and their loved ones to discuss these very personal and somewhat amorphous discussions *outside* of the office, infusion suite or radiation treatment room. *Your acknowledgment goes a long way as the main guide to living with and through cancer. Looking at* My Weekly Recovery Planner *on follow-up visits acknowledges its importance without taking up time.* Your endorsement does not guarantee that each patient will have a long-term survival but opens the possibility that a long-term survival may be possible. Similarly, it will help as the start of a life review for patients with a short life expectancy. Because prediction of survival is so inexact, the planning is helpful, no matter the outcome.

When facing life-threatening illness, patients often become philosophical, asking "Why me?" They are looking for meaning in their suffering and looking for meaning in their lives. Our response as providers is that we "don't know" why one individual develops cancer and another in a similar situation does not. There are other frameworks in which to think about such issues outside of the walls of the office and treatment room.

▩ "STEP IN TO STEP OUT"

The second important function of Living *is to focus on the immediate or "in the now."* Thinking graphically of the typical week of a patient in the midst of chemotherapy, radiation therapy, or combined treatment, the time and effort spent each week on treatment-related activities is considerable, but finite. Traveling to and from treatment, inevitable dwell time in waiting rooms, time with members of your staff, face-to-face provider time, time in the treatment chair, time on the radiation table, imaging, and blood work add up to a solid part of a week. What happens in the rest of the time is quite variable and can be harnessed, at least in part, to good use. How one spends that time is the second important focus of *Living*. Not all of the time needs or should be organized or planned as we often do for our children's free time. Unstructured time can be a valuable resource. For some patients, midlife in careers and child rearing, uncommitted time during treatment may be the most extended period that they have had and can self-program since high school or college.

One of the most useful theoretical structures for clinicians uncomfortable in existential areas has been found in the work of Ludwig and Kabat-Zinn in *Mindfulness in Medicine*.[34,35] With much data being collected about the effects of meditation and relaxation on immune function, endogenous cortisol levels and neurotransmitters, the principles of mindfulness can be a helpful framework to add a comfortable dimension to the patient experience during cancer treatment. Although it has roots in Buddhism and Eastern philosophies, there is a universal quality that is helpful to patients with Judeo-Christian beliefs. However it is packaged, relaxation exercises help someone

The
LEARN
System©

p. 141
My Weekly
Recovery
Planner

for a time to ignore intruding thoughts by focusing on the present and a heightened awareness of time. A sharper focus on the here and now reminds us that each patient is more than just a cancer diagnosis, a footing that is often lost with the fears at diagnosis and through treatment. Concentrating on the experience of living in the moment can foster patience, acceptance, and reduce isolation. It is not an attempt to "fool" oneself to believe that the cancer does not exist, but it encourages, and gives official permission to someone to spend some time *not* thinking about cancer. By doing so, the senses become heightened and thoughts are diverted from the rigors of cancer treatment—for a defined time. Mindfulness focuses one's thoughts on how and what we are doing, or would like to do, in daily life. When combined with progressive relaxation and deep breathing, whether through a physiological mechanism, a psychological one or both, there is a blunting of symptoms, perhaps caused by a change in the way we perceive the symptoms or perhaps a more direct physiologic response mediated by proinflammatory cytokines.

Oncologists' familiarity and skepticism with the processes and purported outcomes in this area feed a schism with those who believe that they are effective without proof. Patients and their caregivers sometimes want to sort out what is fact, which connections may be plausible or are clearly cause–effect relationships, and at times, are outside of our scientific understanding of cancer. The use of these mind–body techniques to prevent cancer or to act as *alternative* treatments in place of standard care is often hard to support. If patients or families describe their use, we do need to know *how* they may be potentially helpful or hurtful. It is important to discern that understanding the techniques is not a religious or spiritual endorsement on a personal level. The use of a mindfulness approach to divert one's attention briefly away from living with cancer is calming, without needing to endorse its spirituality or use to prevent cancer or recurrence. Reinforce the idea that patients who have successfully navigated complicated cancer treatments are well-informed and knowledgeable, but are best not focused on the cancer all the time while neglecting other parts of their lives.

One way to learn about the potential benefits is to try a class in relaxation at a local community organization, outside of the context of cancer. Because the relaxation training is often associated with resistance and flexibility training, there is overlap with another of the LEA**R**N components dealing with **R**est and sleep.

▦ RELY ON OUTSIDE RESOURCES

With our lack of training in these existential and spiritual areas, reaching out to community resources becomes most important. Know who in your community is sensitive to the needs of patients and families with cancer and how they have helped your patients. Help clarify the known limits of mind–body techniques on cancer incidence or recurrence. Be a champion of helpful coping strategies rather than abstaining from discussion if possible.

The role of spirituality in medical treatment in general, and cancer treatment in particular, has been redefined over the last 20 years. As a constitutional concept, *church* has been separated from *state*, but that does not exclude the helpful aspects of spirituality for patients during cancer. The concept has made us so reticent to delve into a characteristic so personal at a time when spirituality could be so helpful. Blind to a particular religious belief, the generic role of spirituality has been brought back into the cancer world through the hospital, and more recently to the ambulatory setting. Seminal work has been done by Laurel Arthur Burton and Reverend George Handzo,[36] with Reverend Handzo being an eminent past director of chaplaincy at Memorial Sloan-Kettering Cancer Center (MSKCC) and now vice president of the Healthcare Chaplaincy Inc., an agency that trains chaplains of many religious backgrounds in clinical pastoral education to serve the ill in the hospital and the community. Reverend Handzo also served to represent pastoral care on the National Comprehensive Cancer Network (NCCN) Distress Management Committee, incorporating the assessment of spirituality and its use in helping patients cope with cancer. Spirituality can help patients come to terms with the existential questions which cancer sparks, such as "Why me?" or the fear that religion may have abandoned them, among other concerns.

Just as generalists in any field have varying skills in specialty work, local ministers may or may not have the special training or skills in pastoral care for cancer patients. Over time, providers and office staff tend to hear from families about which community clergy are particularly helpful. In smaller towns, you will know them yourself.

▦ PRODUCTIVE "BUSYWORK"

Goal-driven patients may seize the opportunity to do something special, or at least plan to do so. Periods of cognitive limitation caused by the sedating effects of antiemetics or analgesics may limit one's ability to work on schedule or complete a project on a narrow timeline. Patients have successfully done something they have longed to do without the chance. The choice of project is determined by educational level, economics, and a host of other demographics. Patients have used technology to learn a language, to play a rudimentary piano, to create computer-assisted design, or to start photography editing. There are many possibilities for patients who are Internet connected. Others may be able to involve in similar activities at no or low cost at local community centers or public libraries. Patients have often said it is hard to read, more so from blurry vision from antiemetics and opioid side effects rather than cognitive impairment. Books on CD or downloaded to an MP3 player can be more suited to the limitations associated with treatment. More than one patient has welcomed the opportunity to revisit the classics she read in high school and college, as she said, "through adult eyes."

Rather than extending the puritanical work ethic, the idea of having something accomplished at the end of the weeks or months in treatment is more appealing to some patients than logging many hours in front of the television.

A chief financial officer of a midsized corporation once joked, "I love game shows. But, how many hours of game shows could *you* watch on television?" Another patient with difficulty sleeping from corticosteroids admitted to more than a few excessive middle-of-the-night purchases on a home shopping channel. He was grateful for being directed to a more goal-driven project. The matriarch of a large multigenerational family was relieved when she was forced to hand over day-to-day responsibility to her daughter and relished a few hours of a personal care aide who visited postoperatively while being treated for a wound infection at home with antibiotics via peripherally inserted central catheter (PICC) line. "This is the first time in my life," she admitted, "Someone is taking care of me for a change."

■ USE THE LEARN SYSTEM TO BRING THEORY TO THE PATIENT EASILY

Whether it is too much daytime television or a little unexpected attention, what is attractive at first may not endure. *My Recovery Plan's "My Weekly Planner"* asks the patient to reevaluate once a week, to keep or shift priorities, and to move on to something else. As treatment progresses and fatigue increases, energy conservation techniques ask the user to set priorities. Having this structure in place will help routinize the time management and help if fatigue sets in.

9

The LEARN System Components: Knowing About Cancer and Its Treatment Eases Uncertainty ("Education")

Health education has become an integral part of medical practice because of the intersection of several forces. With the electronic information explosion, patients and their caregivers access a lot of information of widely varying quality and credibility. In the midst of a consultation or follow-up office visit, it has become impossible to condone, refute, or discuss the merits of the information that is available at the click of a computer mouse. With much of treatment relying on highly technical and complex theory, machinery, and judgment, translating the essence of basic principle and particular details is an ever-growing challenge. It is important to realize that that single office encounter cannot supply enough information for patients and families, unless your practice resembles the idyllic television "Marcus Welby, M.D." type of encounter, with one patient getting seemingly endless attention and thought. This is not a realistic model. Through experience, seasoned providers know that it is often important to clarify points that are *not* posed as questions. Prioritizing information becomes even more of a challenge to anticipate which needs should be addressed.

Through chart audits that confirm mandatory information points to be covered in a patient encounter, having a system to provide reliable information becomes essential to comply with regulatory bodies in that adherence to their rules authorizes us to receive third-party reimbursement. Many practices include a statement with pivotal elements or a summary line in each progress note that acknowledges the educational component of an office or bedside encounter. Such documentation can help meet minimal standards but is most likely just a start.

In the context of cancer survivorship and *My Recovery Plan*, patient education embodies the variety and depth of information that patients and families need to know. That critical mass has outgrown the extent of an office visit. There is help for the individual practitioner. Accessing the skills of your office staff is a "win-win" situation for everyone involved. Your office nurse should have the time and skills to spend some extra moments with patients and families reinforcing concepts you have introduced. A foundation of oncology nursing practice is educational. The Oncology Nursing Society, the major national voice for nurses working in cancer, has dedicated much of their resources to education for patients, families, and its members. Clinical practice resource areas are available for topics related to specific diseases, prevention and detection, professional practice, psychosocial issues, symptom management, treatments, and special populations.[37] Office managers or other office staff can provide much education, however informally, whether teaching about benefits, helping with referrals, or sorting out billing questions. Varying by location and depth of staffing, encouraging staff to develop a list of local resources can add to the job satisfaction and be of inordinate practical help in a smaller practice.

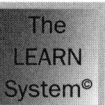

The LEARN System©

p. 141 My Weekly Recovery Planner

Larger treatment centers have made great efforts to write proprietary educational tools and distribute booklets, fact sheets, and information produced by national organizations such as the American Cancer Society, the CancerCare, the National Cancer Institute, the American Society of Clinical Oncology, the American Society for Radiation Oncology, and the Lance Armstrong Foundation. There are many single-disease advocacy organizations that provide excellent patient education materials. Information has been translated into a variety of languages and is available at no or low cost in print, and much can be downloaded from their websites. Collaborating with the hospital where you admit patients avoids duplication of efforts.

Until publications could be easily transmitted online electronically, many larger centers actually wrote and produced their own booklets and pamphlets. With the increasing costs of printing and a constantly evolving knowledge base, reliance on national resources has intensified. The technological age has made current information easily available to patients at both larger centers and smaller practices.

WHAT PATIENTS AND FAMILIES NEED TO KNOW AND DO

The backbone of *My Recovery Plan* and *Learn to Live Through Cancer: What You Need to Know and Do* is educational in the fullest sense. How much patients and families need to know (and do) and at when it needs to be discussed varies, owed to several factors.

A fine balance exists to determine what and how much information to provide to patients and families as well as when to discuss it. Outside of the arena of clinical trials, such information is not tracked, and varies quite a bit over settings, patients, and providers. Medical providers often make a global overall and quick assessment of how much information a patient and family can absorb. It is well accepted that patients retain about half or less of the information provided. The ability to retain vital information is affected by many variables: type of cancer, preexisting cognitive impairments, level of fear, anxiety, or sadness. Knowing that many or even most patients admit to feeling "numb" when they first learn of their diagnosis, that natural reaction serves as an obstacle to absorb, process, and retain information related to their cancer and the proposed treatment.

Beyond printed material, patients and families have other concerns, some of which are personal. Information on websites and in brochures may or may not apply to each individual, or if does apply, some folks believe it is "for someone else." This void in the information chain is sometimes filled by support groups. However, with the information explosion that is carried right into one's home, there is less of an impetus to join a support group than there was in the past. Although not the same as "being there," the personal connection that participants make can be experienced on the phone and through the keyboard, providing that a patient and family participate in some medium.

Dr. Carolyn Messner, director of education at CancerCare corroborates this trend (personal communication, March 2011). She says,

Face-to-face group interest has declined at CancerCare as well as nationally due to cancer patients' and survivors' busy schedules, inability to take time off from work, or other activities for the added travel time involved in a face-to-face group. We currently offer 25 different online groups and many telephone support groups. We do offer face-to-face groups but fewer of them. We also want to include all of our rural patients for whom travel involves hundreds of miles. And the great appeal of our teleconference programs is the ease of participation.

The array of educational talks in real time, on the telephone, that include questions and answers, with the further options of listening again on podcast and e-mailing questions is astounding. In March 2011, 83 podcasts covering a variety of topics were accessible online on Cancer*Care*'s website (http://www.cancercare.org). A combined effort of the Wellness Community and Gilda's Club covered some of the same topics, as have some others.* Livestrong.org features videos as well as survivor interviews online. The National Cancer Institute offers written online information as well (http://www.cancer.org).

It's impossible to keep track of the many community resources out there. An informed oncology social worker at your local cancer center or at your chapter of the American Cancer Society does so. Training for the Patient Navigator Program offered by area offices of the American Cancer Society recommends good and up-to-date educational tools for your patients. Your office's role is to strongly encourage patients and families to link to them. That can be done with simple brochures in your waiting room, or charging your receptionist or office manager with the responsibility of giving the information to each new patient. If there is no "local" oncology social worker in your community, or for patients who prefer the connection on the telephone, Cancer*Care* services, including telephone service to patients and families *at no charge* via toll free numbers (1-800-813-HOPE for patients and families who find telephone access easier than online). A full list of resources is available in the Patient and Family Worksheets section.

Colleagues have often wondered what gets discussed at support groups, and some volunteer to attend sessions whereas others invited guests who speak about a topic or answer questions. During these support group meetings, some staff reviews are inevitably traded (for the good *or* bad), but the bulk of time and effort is devoted to sharing information and experiences. Having another patient or family acknowledge an experience gives a sense of validation and understanding. Learning from someone who is a few steps ahead can also be helpful for practical as well as emotional issues. There is a dimension of camaraderie that veteran patients provide and professionals cannot fulfill. Support groups are sometimes time limited or ongoing, and either involve patients with the same type of cancer or treatment, or mix these factors. At times, part of patients' or caregivers' reticence is that other patients may be "too sick," or that they may die during the weeks that the group runs, and such an event is easily personalized. Perhaps the hardest and most rewarding discussions in support groups force patients to acknowledge on a personal level what providers see over the course of their career when a patient has progressive disease and dies. At times, patients or caregivers refuse to go back. Other times, it is the experience in the group that serves as the motivation to have a serious discussion with family members or providers.

---

* I have been a consultant to Cancer*Care* from 1985 through 2005 and have served on the original Medical Advisory Board of Gilda's Club for the New York center.

▓ PATIENTS WANT US TO KNOW

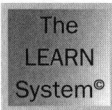

The
LEARN
System©

p. 140
Questions
I Want
Answered

Patients want us to acknowledge that cancer changes their lives, and that the experience can force a new life outlook that takes less for granted. Things that were trivial or nuisances before may become even more trivial with cancer lurking, and that translates into being less tolerant about incidentals such as waiting in line, traffic jams, and the many other "uncontrollables" of daily life. Patients often don't want us providers to know how afraid they are and how the has changed their "center of gravity." A list of questions heard over the years is included in the subsequent box and in *Questions I Want Answered*.

What is cancer?

Why me?

How did I get it?

Why didn't I know about it sooner?

How do I find out what type of cancer it is and what treatment I need?

What is the stage and type?

Will this kill me?

How much time do I have?

Can it be cured? . . . controlled? . . . put in remission?

How will I feel?

Will I recover and be myself?

What will the treatment include?

Can I continue to work?

How can I arrange for a second opinion? (No offense, please. But this is serious and I need to know.)

Who can help with my kids? Will I need help at home?

What do I need to do during my treatment? Eat, exercise?

What will be affected by the cancer and by the treatments?

What about vitamins and supplements?

What are "clinical trials"?

What is important to me now?

What do I have to do to get better?

When will I feel okay again? Will I be the same?

Will the cancer come back?

continued

continued

Is it familial?

What do my family and friends need to know?

Will I be able to forget all of what is happening?

How long will I need follow-up care? What will it be?

Will I be okay?

What if nothing works?

What will happen if I get sicker?

Will you stick by me if treatment does not work?

How . . . and when will I die?

No provider is expected to know or supply answers to all of these questions, especially all at once. Some of the answers are not really known, but the curiosity still exists. Some have no true right answer but are very personal in nature. It is unlikely that you will get to know your patients well enough at least at the start of treatment to know *how* they go about their daily lives, how they best process information, or if they discuss feelings easily or are more stoic. One of the advantages of using *My Recovery Plan* is that these issues, as tough as they are, become explicitly discussed.

The two cases highlighted in the "Education" section of *Learn to Live Through Cancer* demonstrate two scenarios common to newly diagnosed patients. One is a situation in which a concerned family, believing it is necessary to *discuss* feelings, hopes that a stoic patient rather suddenly becomes someone who discusses his feelings easily. The second case highlights another apprehensive family who believes that a patient must be "happy" to prolong his survival and maximize treatment efficacy.

Beyond outlining the usual and expected information that patients and families need to navigate, some solutions are suggested. Telephone or Internet support groups are only attractive to a subgroup. Educational activities in-person, on the telephone, or online have some of the same benefits. Individual or family counseling, face to face or on the telephone or online is another option. Collecting information via brochures, books, or online can fill part of the education gap. Informal discussion in waiting rooms brings camaraderie and information, although not all of the information is always accurate.

■ CONTENT AREAS OF SPECIAL INTEREST

Certain areas of supportive care can and do fill textbooks and trade books written for and sold to the general public. The LEARN System components include most of them, which are related to rest, activity, nutrition, and how one lives life while being treated for cancer, or *living through cancer*. Some areas of interest do not fall under these categories. Because they are discussed in *Learn to Live Through Cancer: What You Need to Know and Do*, they are listed here to avoid "surprise" mentions by patients and families using the guide.

- *Pharmacological Approaches to Pain*, focusing on basic guideline to assess pain and use a stepwise opioid family-based approach, respecting half-lives of drugs, striving to simplify dosing schedules using long-acting or time-release preparations, maximizing the use of adjuvant analgesics and nonpharmacologic approaches.

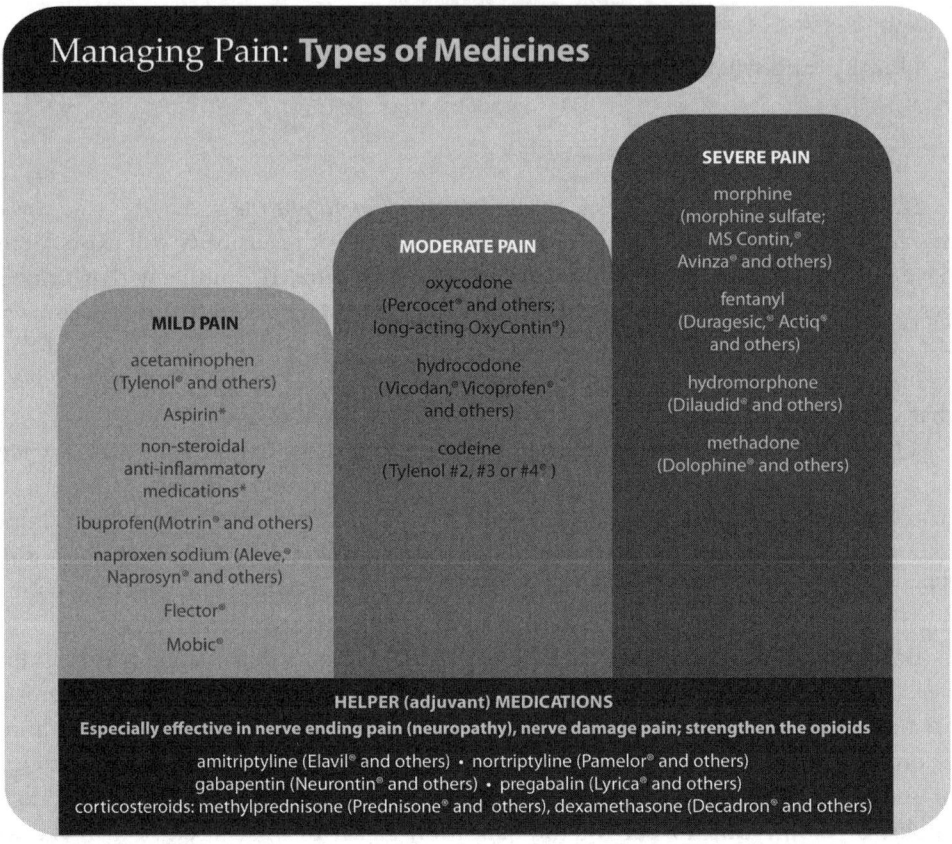

Managing Pain: **Types of Medicines**

SEVERE PAIN

morphine
(morphine sulfate;
MS Contin,®
Avinza® and others)

fentanyl
(Duragesic,® Actiq®
and others)

hydromorphone
(Dilaudid® and others)

methadone
(Dolophine® and others)

MODERATE PAIN

oxycodone
(Percocet® and others;
long-acting OxyContin®)

hydrocodone
(Vicodan,® Vicoprofen®
and others)

codeine
(Tylenol #2, #3 or #4®)

MILD PAIN

acetaminophen
(Tylenol® and others)

Aspirin*

non-steroidal
anti-inflammatory
medications*

ibuprofen(Motrin® and others)

naproxen sodium (Aleve,®
Naprosyn® and others)

Flector®

Mobic®

HELPER (adjuvant) MEDICATIONS
Especially effective in nerve ending pain (neuropathy), nerve damage pain; strengthen the opioids

amitriptyline (Elavil® and others) · nortriptyline (Pamelor® and others)
gabapentin (Neurontin® and others) · pregabalin (Lyrica® and others)
corticosteroids: methylprednisone (Prednisone® and others), dexamethasone (Decadron® and others)

*Use with care during chemotherapy and radiation therapy to avoid changes in blood clotting.

- *Antiemetics*, because many of the regimens use *prn* dosing, quite a bit of familiarity is needed by the patient and family. Also, a drug family-based system, this graphic has been helpful to patients and families.

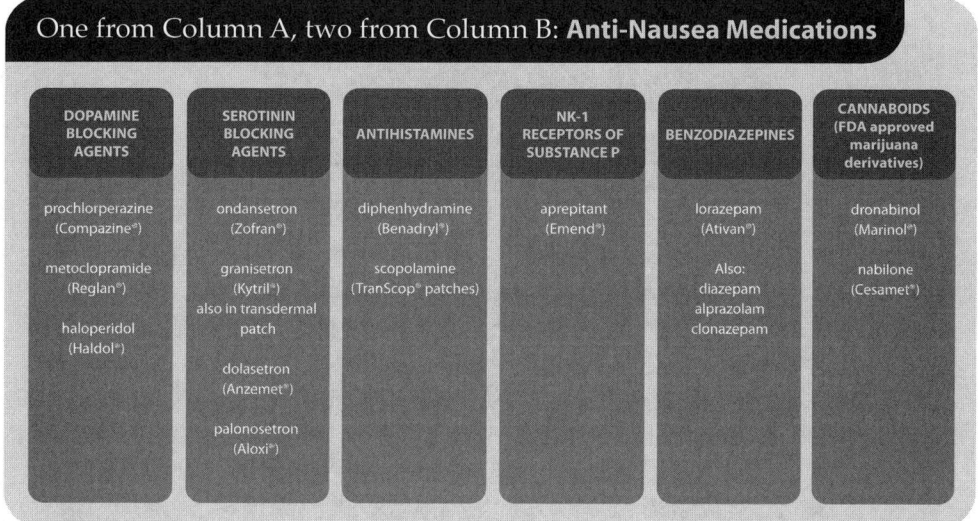

One from Column A, two from Column B: **Anti-Nausea Medications**

DOPAMINE BLOCKING AGENTS	SEROTININ BLOCKING AGENTS	ANTIHISTAMINES	NK-1 RECEPTORS OF SUBSTANCE P	BENZODIAZEPINES	CANNABOIDS (FDA approved marijuana derivatives)
prochlorperazine (Compazine®)	ondansetron (Zofran®)	diphenhydramine (Benadryl®)	aprepitant (Emend®)	lorazepam (Ativan®)	dronabinol (Marinol®)
metoclopramide (Reglan®)	granisetron (Kytril®) also in transdermal patch	scopolamine (TranScop® patches)		Also: diazepam alprazolam clonazepam	nabilone (Cesamet®)
haloperidol (Haldol®)	dolasetron (Anzemet®)				
	palonosetron (Aloxi®)				

Nausea experienced during chemotherapy is often managed using one, or a combination, of any of the medications listed above.

- *Constipation Ladder*, employing a ladder analogy to work from fluid and fiber through enemas.

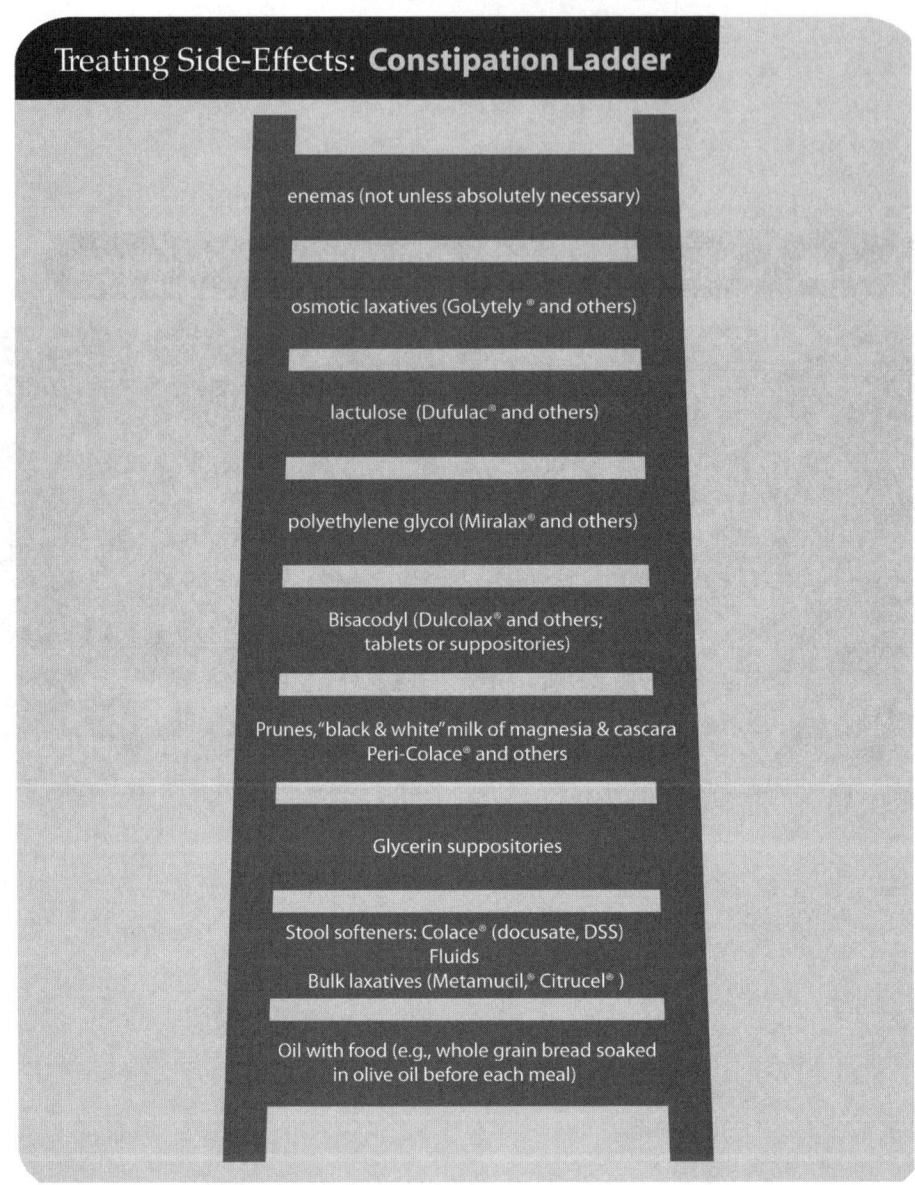

Treating Side-Effects: **Constipation Ladder**

enemas (not unless absolutely necessary)

osmotic laxatives (GoLytely ® and others)

lactulose (Dufulac® and others)

polyethylene glycol (Miralax® and others)

Bisacodyl (Dulcolax® and others; tablets or suppositories)

Prunes, "black & white" milk of magnesia & cascara Peri-Colace® and others

Glycerin suppositories

Stool softeners: Colace® (docusate, DSS)
Fluids
Bulk laxatives (Metamucil,® Citrucel®)

Oil with food (e.g., whole grain bread soaked in olive oil before each meal)

Start at bottom of ladder, increasing dose if necessary. When maximum dose is reached, move to the treatment option one step up on the ladder. Continue up the ladder as each maximum dose and desired effect is achieved.

- *Diarrhea Ladder*, conceptually consistent with the constipation ladder, moving from the least noxious treatments to the most up the ladder.

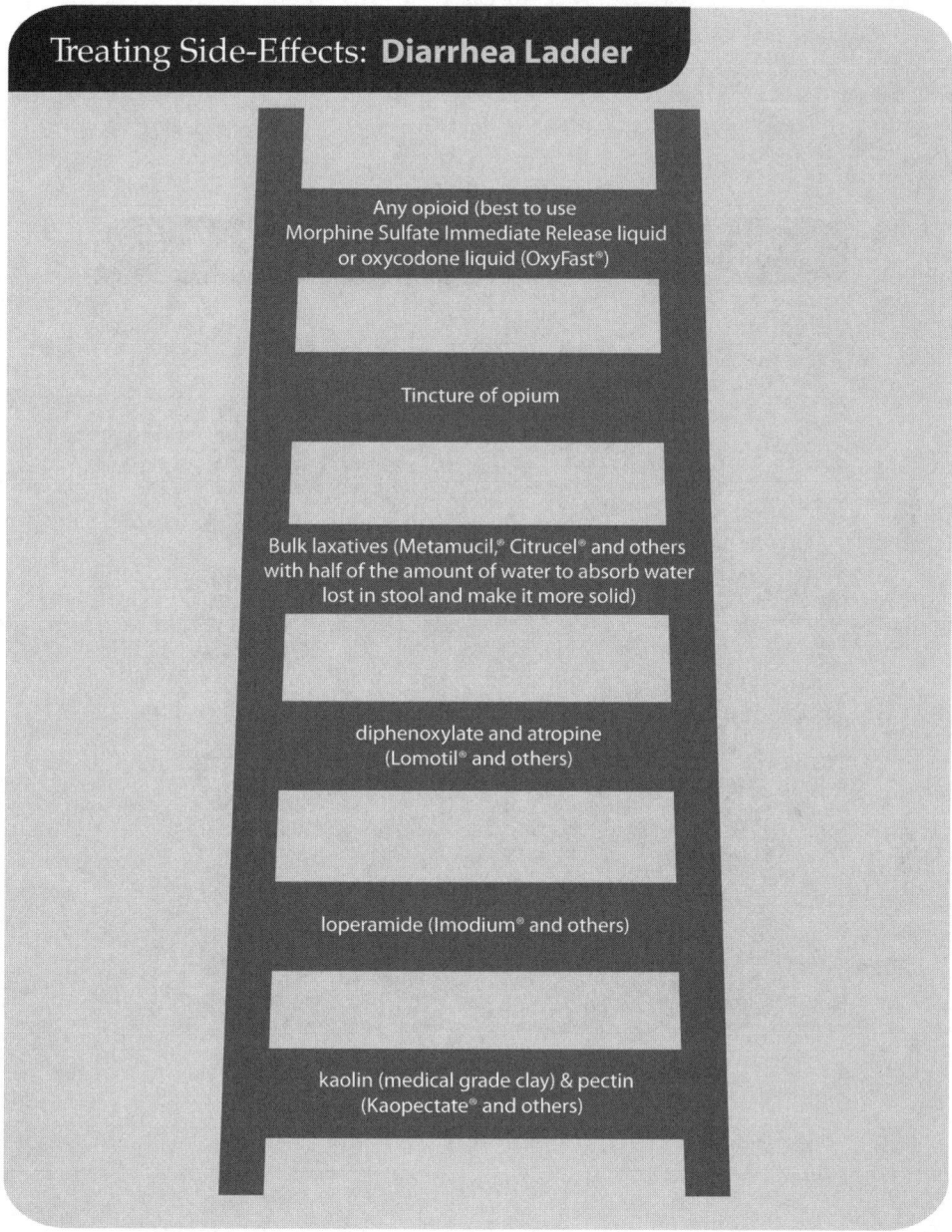

Treating Side-Effects: **Diarrhea Ladder**

Any opioid (best to use Morphine Sulfate Immediate Release liquid or oxycodone liquid (OxyFast®)

Tincture of opium

Bulk laxatives (Metamucil,® Citrucel® and others with half of the amount of water to absorb water lost in stool and make it more solid)

diphenoxylate and atropine (Lomotil® and others)

loperamide (Imodium® and others)

kaolin (medical grade clay) & pectin (Kaopectate® and others)

Start at bottom of ladder, increasing dose if necessary. When maximum dose is reached, move to the treatment option one step up on the ladder. Continue up the ladder as each maximum dose is reached.

- *The Rules* based on a common paradigm, useful to sort out cancer-related developments that need medical evaluation from those that are rites of passage in virtually every survivor.

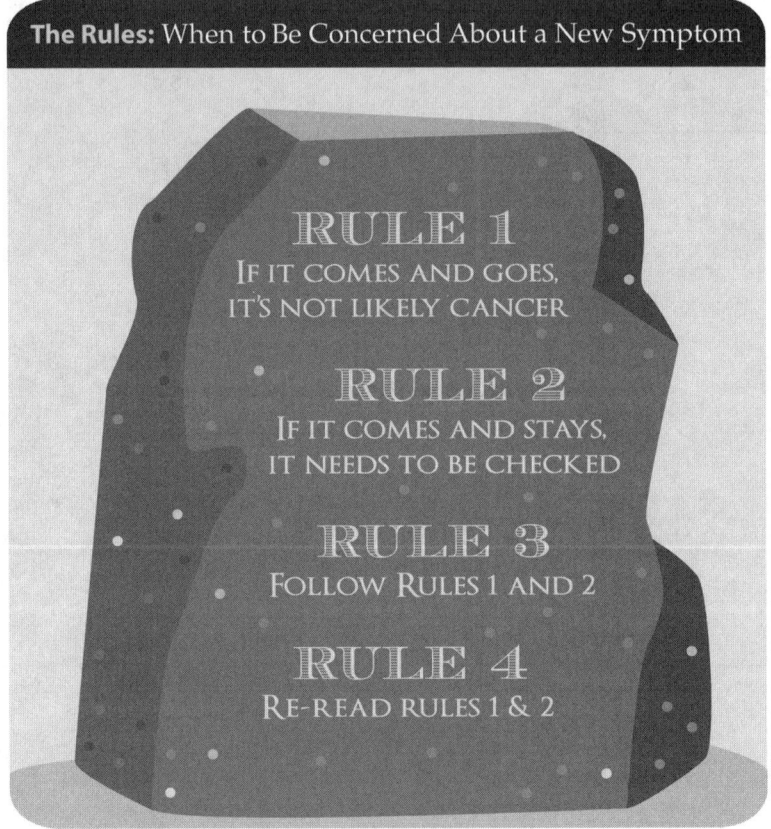

▩ EXTRA WORK

A potential criticism of *My Recovery Plan* using *The LEARN System* is that it is a lot of work. Some of the efforts are directed to gaining good cancer information and a better understanding of what it is like to have a life-threatening illness with an extended period of treatment and a lot of uncertainty. One could think that the extra work—self-assessment questionnaires and form completion—is simply a sophisticated form of diversion to keep patients and families so busy that they do not feel frightened and isolated, or believing that they are the only ones in such a situation. There are other more entertaining forms of diversion available, and they are suggested in this book as well, elevating these educational activities to a higher purpose.

Following the professional credo, "see one, do one, teach one," patients are encouraged to *give forward* in an effort to help others while they are coming to terms with their own illness and treatment. Giving *forward* is a progressive version of giving *back* in which you help the next generation of patients and families. It can be financial or time-based or both, or formal or informal. Virtually, everyone knows someone who is being treated for cancer. Giving forward can be as simple as making a meal for someone in your community or driving a patient to and from a follow-up appointment. The choices are vast.

10

The LEARN System Components: Maintaining Activity During Treatment Improves Outcomes ("**A**ctivity" and Exercise)

Few of us embrace the concept of personal exercise goals easily. In a 2010 survey by Karvinen and colleagues,[38] 64% of respondents (N = 199; 30% of 702 sample) inquired about their patients' physical activity on some or most visits. Even when the question is asked, having some follow-up suggestions will encourage the patient to incorporate activity into their daily routine.

The American College of Sports Medicine[39] held a round table in 2009 to discuss guidelines for cancer survivors. Historically, clinicians advised patients with cancer to rest and to avoid activity; however, emerging research on exercise has challenged this recommendation. The round table concluded that exercise training is safe during and after cancer treatments and results in improvements in physical functioning, quality of life (QoL), and cancer-related fatigue in several cancer survivor groups. The full implications for disease outcomes and survival are still to be discovered. Nevertheless, the benefits to physical functioning and QoL are sufficient for the recommendation that cancer survivors follow the *2008 Physical Activity Guidelines for Americans*, with specific exercise programming adaptations based on disease and treatment-related adverse effects. These guidelines are directed at the healthy American population, not at patients with cancer. The advice to "avoid inactivity," even in cancer patients with existing disease or undergoing difficult treatments, is most likely helpful.

▪ A GROWING EVIDENCE BASE

Pekmezi and Demark-Wahnefried[40] reviewed 21 randomized clinical trials *suggesting* that physical activity interventions are safe for cancer survivors and produce improvements in fitness, strength, and physical function. Additionally, there may be improvements in biomarkers (insulin levels, insulin-like growth factors, oxidative DNA damage, tumor proliferation rates) and overall survival.

Clinicians currently allude to a tailored dose of activity at every phase of treatment, informally and intuitively. Think about the usual advice postoperatively for, virtually, any cancer surgery: "Be sure to dangle your legs off the bed today," followed by "The nurse will get you into a chair this afternoon," then "Be sure to walk up and down the hallway today even if you push your IV pole around." Before discharge, that may be the very last directive on activity one gets. Directions for patients and families can be more consistent at discharge and beyond, especially with hospital stays being so much shorter than ever. Rarely do practices *routinely* refer patients to physical therapy or for a physical medicine and rehabilitation (PM&R) consult in order to customize an activity program to specific clinical needs.

▨ BARRIERS TO RECOMMENDATION OF PHYSICAL ACTIVITY

A few barriers exist that discourage any formal recommendation for activity before, during, and after cancer treatment. Karvinen et al[38] identified the lack of time during consultation or office visit, the lack of clarity in recommendations, concerns about the safety of activity, concerns about the effectiveness of physical activity, a lack of patient interest, and a lack of reimbursement for counseling about physical activity tailored to a patient's specific clinical situation.

Clarkson and Kaufman[41] have brought forth a theoretical concern with breast cancer in response to strenuous resistance exercise. Muscle satellite (progenitor) cells are activated to reenter the cell cycle and proliferate. Satellite cells are a type of adult stem cells that can become myocytes, adipocytes, or osteocytes. By becoming myocytes, satellite cells help to repair injured muscle. Satellite cells do not divide as rapidly in older animals, and as a result, muscles do not heal as rapidly as humans and animals age. Satellite cells can then contribute their nuclear material into the fiber to facilitate muscle repair, regeneration, and hypertrophy. Cancer therapy damages rapidly dividing cells and thus has the potential to target satellite cells that enter into the cell cycle. Although satellite cells are self-renewing, they are not completely replenished over the life span, so losses in this progenitor population via resistance exercise and cancer therapy may impair the maintenance of muscle mass with aging. The researchers advise that before recommending resistance training during breast cancer treatment, we must have more information about cancer treatment effects on activated satellite cells in human studies.

Based on most current information, our patients can benefit from a bit more direction. Safety, as a prime goal of patients and providers alike, is a paramount factor. However, there are simple activities that patients can do at home requiring little equipment, expense, or risk.

Following is a generic simple activity algorithm. Of course, it needs to be personalized to type and stage of cancer, type of treatment being given, comorbidities, and general physical condition prior to (and during) cancer treatment.

Simple Activity Algorithm (Until Formal Physical Medicine and Rehabilitation or Physical Therapy Evaluation)

Inpatient Post-op: Dangle legs from bed → sit in bedside chair → range of motion movements in bed or chair → walk in hallways (with or without assistance) → physical medicine and rehabilitation (PM&R) evaluation or physical therapy consult

continued

> ### Simple Activity Algorithm (Until Formal Physical Medicine and Rehabilitation or Physical Therapy Evaluation)
>
> *continued*
>
> **Home (ambulatory):** Make sure to get up to go to bathroom (with or without assistance) q XX hours → walk around on one level at home → walk a little farther and longer each day (if in single family home, begin steps slowly, increasing number of times walking up and down a flight of steps; if in apartment house: walk around in hallways → use stairs or fire stairs when not in use by others, from qd to bid to tid → if weather is favorable, walk outside to mailbox, get newspaper, increasing length and duration of walk. If able, go to indoor shopping mall before 9 AM (or similar surroundings) where it is climate controlled and unobstructed. → Arrange for ambulatory physical therapy or PM&R consult to prescription (Rx) resistance and stretching components of routine.
>
> **Home (bedbound):** Range of motion movements with assistance if necessary.

An ideal plan for physical activity is best designed with the patient himself or herself, taking many factors into account. Three types of activity should be included as tolerated and tailored to the patient's abilities: *increasing endurance*, *adding resistance* to maximize lean body mass, and *retain flexibility*. To avoid falls and transfer without incident from bed to chair to toilet and shower, activities that reinforce stability are also important. Aerobic activity that puts the pulse to 150% of a resting pulse may be harder to achieve, with energy limitations or comorbidities. It may spend too much precious energy and may be contraindicated. But alternatives such as gentle movement in a recumbent bike or "chair aerobics" or using devices such as elastic bands or other devices can increase heart rate in a controlled way to much lower levels. Expert instruction about the safe use of these devices is critical.

During a formal consult, the expert will advise the patient and family and personalize the plan, particularly with respect to mode of activity, intensity of activity, and frequency. Such a customized approach is designed to avoid any skeletal-related event or other untoward side effects.

> ### Components of *Activity*
>
> *Aerobic* activity with increase in heart rate
>
> Activity that enhances *endurance* by adding resistance
>
> Maintaining *flexibility*

The expected outcomes of physical activity include a better appetite, a more restorative sleep, weight control, and protection against falls. Additionally, there should be a counterintuitive reduction in fatigue and an easier recovery from treatments. In a noncancer

Activity in METs (Metabolic Equivalent of Tasks)	
Physical Activity	**MET**
Light Intensity Activities	< 3
sleeping	0.9
watching television	1.0
writing, desk work, typing	1.8
walking, less than 2.0 mph (3.2 km/h), level ground, strolling, very slow	2.0
Moderate Intensity Activities	3 to 6
bicycling, stationary, 50 watts, very light effort	3.0
calisthenics, home exercise, light or moderate effort, general	3.5
bicycling, <10 mph (16 km/h), leisure, to work or for pleasure	4.0
bicycling, stationary, 100 watts, light effort	5.5
Vigorous Intensity Activities	> 6
jogging, general	7.0
calisthenics (e.g., push-ups, sit-ups, pull-ups, jumping jacks), heavy, vigorous effort	8.0
running, jogging, in place	8.0
rope jumping	10.0

population, there is continued inquiry into the mechanism through which physical activity translates into psychological well-being. Both the endorphin and endocannabinoid systems are thought to be responsible for the "feel good" after physical activity. Whether directly caused by a sense of accomplishment in an activity not usually associated with cancer therapies or indirectly caused by an effect via neurotransmitters, a reduction in anxiety and maintenance of self-esteem are also reasonably expected outcomes.

With physical activity measured in metabolic equivalent of tasks (METs), a general list to discourage a "too much too soon" approach is included in *Learn to Live Through Cancer: What You Need to Know and Do*.

■ WHAT ARE THE PRACTICAL BENEFITS OF INCREASED PHYSICAL ACTIVITY DURING CANCER TREATMENT?

Muscle atrophy can be prevented by movement, and disuse can lead to atrophy. Stretching and flexing muscles help avoid skeletal muscle hypodynamia and improve muscle strength and cardiopulmonary function.

Jones and colleagues[42] looked at the benefits of exercise at key points in treatment and survivorship: preoperative, postoperative during adjuvant treatment, and following the completion of primary therapy and palliation. They conclude that the current evidence base provides strong, however preliminary, evidence that exercise therapy is well tolerated and safe. Exercise at key points can mitigate several common treatment-related side effects with early disease both during and after adjuvant therapy.

It can be assumed that investigation into the restorative power of exercise for patients with cancer has lagged behind applications to other illnesses because of a perception that patients with cancer are unable to participate or have a period of survival, that is too short to warrant the effort. The use of exercise to extend survival remains questionable even today; however, such doubt cannot nullify the beneficial effects on QoL and symptom control.

Preoperative studies encompassing either aerobic training, resistance training, or a combination of the two, three times a week for 30 to 60 minutes over 2 to 24 weeks, showed improvements in muscular strength, cardiorespiratory fitness, functional QoL, fatigue, anxiety, and self-esteem with few adverse events.[43] Pooled data indicated that exercise training was associated with a statistically significant increase in $\dot{V}o_2$ (peak volume of oxygen consumption) with minimal adverse events.

Reported during treatment for breast cancer or non–small-cell lung cancer, exercise may still reduce treatment-related side effects and is well tolerated, although it may show less of an effect than afterward. The effect of exercise on survival is harder to show across the board but it is thought to be beneficial.[44] Its effect varies by type of cancer and amount of physical activity but is not associated with negative outcomes. The National Cancer Institute of Canada is sponsoring the phase III trial, Colon Health and Life-Long Exercise Change (CHALLENGE), investigating the effects of regular exercise on recurrence and cancer-specific mortality in colorectal patients with cancer.

With progressive disease, patients may have a higher relative benefit from exercise-based interventions where the improvements in QoL are the main goals of care. Such a finding has been harder to ascertain because of a dearth of clinical trials and interest until quite recently.

▉ MORE OF THE *COMMON SENSE* APPROACH

In view of the promising but limited knowledge about the specific effects of activity during the various phases of cancer treatment and the differences in patients with cancers of different types and stages, it is persuasive to include a recommendation for a tailored level of activity from the time of diagnosis through survivorship with either stable or progressive disease. A reduction in symptom burden and improvements in QoL have been consistent over the only very recent burgeoning number of studies. Following the usual clinical mantra to assess and reevaluate patients throughout their care, including some activity as part of a treatment plan can be easily monitored for adverse events during a routine follow-up visit. The *My Weekly Planner* form can be visually scanned at follow-up visits for oversight of adverse outcomes. In the A or Activity box, patients and/or their designee summarize what

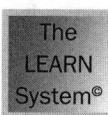

The LEARN System©

p. 141 My Weekly Recovery Planner

they have learned and done during the week. Such screening information can serve as a reminder to trigger the referral to the physical therapist or PM&R specialist for consult and allow you to see the results of their recommendations after the PM&R visits have been made.

▓ ACTIVITY: A VITAL TOOL TO COMBAT FATIGUE

The symptom of fatigue straddles each of the LEARN categories in *My Recovery Plan* because it is so closely interrelated to each of the other components of nutrition and rest. Fatigue is a multidetermined symptom, related to one's attitude and outlook (part of the L [Living] and E [Education component]), how active one is (A), the quality and amount of rest (R) achieved, and nutritional state (N).

The problem of fatigue rose prominently in the consciousness of the cancer community in the 1990s with the marketing of erythropoietin products. Because of their connection to cancer-induced and cancer-associated factors mediated by anemia, an approved and successful treatment for anemia became a natural avenue to highlight fatigue in QoL during cancer treatment.

Although fatigue is a very common symptom during cancer, it had previously been underestimated and poorly understood. No matter which symptom burden scale is used, fatigue is one of the top five symptoms reported by patients. Fatigue is listed as a potential side effect for most cytotoxic chemotherapies, is commonly experienced by patients receiving radiation therapy, and is related to the suppression of both estrogen and testosterone in women and men. Prior to raising both patient and provider awareness of fatigue, it was so prevalent and commonplace that fatigue was accepted as a routine part of cancer that needed to be endured. Minimizing or eliminating it was rarely addressed.

Although suggesting an aliquot of physical activity to combat fatigue is counterintuitive, it is a foundation to the multifaceted management of this distressing symptom.

▓ DIFFERENTIAL DIAGNOSIS OF FATIGUE

The causes of fatigue can be best compartmentalized into two categories: cancer-*induced* and cancer-*associated*. This dichotomy (borrowed from weight loss models) helps in easily thinking through a differential diagnosis and management.

Sorting out the causes of fatigue will help sort out the management issues quickly. Patients who consider themselves frail or whose diagnosis is preceded by a downward course of reduced daily activities—homebound or bedbound—are starting out with fewer energy stores and less of an energy reserve on which to fall back. Correction of whichever factors are *associated* with fatigue may relieve all or part of the symptoms, when such an intervention is possible. Sorting out medications, checking thyroid function, and evaluating for infection or undue distress are possible. Replacement of estrogen or testosterone in hormonally dependent cancers may not be prudent. *l*-Carnitine is a micronutrient that may contribute to fatigue and its replacement can benefit some patients.[45]

Causes of Cancer-Associated Fatigue	Causes of Cancer-Induced Fatigue
Preexisting Debility	**Hypermetabolic State**
Pain	Anemia
Sleep changes	Cachexia
Distress	Cytokine effects on CNS
Infection	Disease progression
Hypothyroidism	
Estrogen or testosterone suppression	
Organ dysfunction:	
Heart—poor perfusion	
Lungs—hypoxia	
Liver failure	
Kidney failure	
Brain and spinal cord	
Hyperglycemia	
Sedating medications	
Occult alcohol or drug use	
Hypercalcemia	

Abbreviation: CNS, central nervous system.

■ CANCER-*INDUCED* FATIGUE IS MORE THAN JUST BEING TIRED

The eloquent words that patients use to describe cancer-induced fatigue tip us off that the condition is serious. The feeling has been described as an overwhelming sense of tiredness at rest, exhaustion with activity, a lack of energy that precludes daily tasks, an inertia or lack of endurance, and the loss of vigor.[46] The depth in the frustration that is expressed when patients want desperately to function at their preillness levels is astounding.

In their comprehensive review of the mechanisms of fatigue in a variety of chronic illnesses, Davis and Walsh[46] shed confirmatory light on the origin of fatigue in cancer as being mediated centrally, extrapolating from animal data using both electroencephalography and peripheral electromyography. Inagaki and colleagues[47] correlated plasma interleukin 6 levels with the physical subscale score of the Cancer Fatigue Scale. With interleukin 6's prominently suspected role in cancer-induced cachexia, evidence further points to its role in the debility that arises from cancer and treatment.

If fatigue is mostly centrally mediated, with multiple factors that augment it, The LEARN System's selection of components hit those factors directly to diminish the symptoms as an adjunct to identifying a compound fighting the proinflammatory cytokine itself.

▦ WORKUP OF FATIGUE

In the absence of a specialist whose main clinical focus is to diagnose and treat cancer-related fatigue, an office-based workup can be easily done. Many of the tests needed are done for most patients undergoing treatment.

Targeted Office-Based Workup of Fatigue in Cancer

History:
- Exact list of mediations: current, recently stopped
- *Candid* mention of alcohol or drugs (not acquired by your Rx)

Exam:
- Strength of peripheral muscles in arms, legs
- Overall sense of progressive disease: pallor, weight loss, loss of skeletal muscle
- Bleeding or infection: hematomas, petechiae, fever
- Focal bone pain

Blood work:
- Complete blood count (CBC; to rule out anemia, infection)
- Thyroid-stimulating hormone (TSH; to rule out hypothyroidism, especially after head/neck or chest radiation therapy)
- Metabolic profile (calcium, magnesium, glycemic control, kidney, liver function)

Imaging (likely recently done)
Electrocardiogram (EKG)

A 58-year-old wife of a nurse practitioner had been a survivor of fallopian tube cancer for 7 years. She had a total abdominal hysterectomy and bilateral salpingo-oophorectomy (TAH/BSO), systemic treatment with paclitaxel and carboplatinum, and local treatment of paclitaxel through an intraperitoneal shunt. Since the treatment ended, she has never regained her precancer energy and sense of strength. She has remained as active as possible in her work and family activities, and prides herself about never missing a major school event or milestone in her children's development, despite her lengthy treatment. In the last 3 months, she has been tired and has to "push myself even more than usual" to maintain her work and family activities. She feels her gym workout takes too much energy without benefit and says she feels less steady than usual on the treadmill. Her weight has been stable, exactly at her ideal body weight, and her body mass index (BMI) = 22. Having just returned from a family vacation, she reports feeling "wonderfully restored but still as tired as I can imagine."

With stable imaging, complete blood count (CBC), metabolic profile and thyroid-stimulating hormone (TSH) close to within normal limits (WNL), stable tumor markers, and no medication changes, her case was perplexing until her gynecologic oncologist suggested an *anti-Yo antibody*. During the time the results were pending, further unsteadiness became evident in everyday activities, more than just at the gym. An abnormal *anti-Yo* titer best established that the fatigue was a hidden sign of recurrence, and she was referred for intravenous gamma globulin with a stabilization of symptoms. The fatigue was the defining symptom that established the diagnosis of a recurrence.

FATIGUE AFTER CANCER TREATMENT

Even patients who will invest short-term comfort for the chance of extended survival become frustrated when fatigue remains months or years after successful treatment. In a literature review, Harrington and colleagues[48] found consistent reports of burdensome symptoms in survivors of breast, gynecological, prostate, and colorectal cancers with physical and cognitive limitations, depression/anxiety, sleep problems, fatigue, pain, and sexual dysfunction reported more than 10 years following treatment. Although there are very few studies showing that a preventive intervention can avoid persistent symptoms, patients seem reticent to describe the symptom burden while experiencing the gratitude of being alive. A small randomized exercise adherence study of 41 sedentary women with early stage breast cancer receiving hormonal therapies showed improvements in physical activity, strength, central adiposity, and social well-being with lower extremity function benefits, but extended only 3 months.[49] Lack of workplace accommodation was significantly related to fatigue at 18-month follow-up in the Netherlands.[50]

SYMPTOMATIC TREATMENT OF FATIGUE

Optimal management of fatigue, based on current knowledge, involves a multidisciplinary approach. Involvement of a PM&R specialist and/or physical therapist, oncology nutritionist or registered dietician, and education from an oncology nurse is all best reinforced by you. Reinforcement of the efforts by a psychosocial counselor can strengthen the message and relieve some of the burden on a busy oncologist.

Energy conservation is another technique that is partly intuitive, but for many patients, this needs to be made explicit. The National Comprehensive Cancer Network (NCCN), "NCCN Clinical Guidelines in Oncology: Cancer-Related Fatigue V.1.2011,"[51] best summarize the basic principles: set priorities (do what is valued first), pace oneself, delegate tasks when possible, schedule activities at the times of day when energy level peaks, use labor-assisting devices (e.g., wheelchairs, walkers, commodes), eliminate nonessential activities, structured daily routine, attend to one activity at a time, and use distraction.

Commonly conceived as *comfort* measures, massage and stretching can be of great relief. Whether stretching and resistance training is packaged as *yoga* or under some other name, it depends on your community's understanding and familiarity with yoga. But the principles remain sound, even when described by less misunderstood terminology. A growing minority of insurance carriers reimburse for massage or stretching/resistance training beyond physical therapy benefits, although that trend is changing because these modalities are sometimes bundled under a *wellness* benefit for general health maintenance.

The use of stimulant medications can be quite helpful as a symptomatic treatment in its most classic sense. Stimulants do not treat the cause, but can be of significant help in minimizing the symptom of fatigue.

Stimulants were first used in cancer for patients receiving significant analgesia from opioids with concomitant sedation. Stimulants helped offset the sedation without adding extra pain relief, but allowed a patient to take higher doses of opioids while being alert enough to participate in daily activities. Later studies identified that stimulants can also potentiate the analgesic effects of opioids.[52] Subsequently, stimulants were found to have direct adjuvant properties as analgesics.[53] Stimulants have also been prescribed to enhance and lift mood as an alternative to waiting for the lag time in the action of antidepressants in cancer and noncancer patients.

Having a tainted history, stimulants such as dextroamphetamine are less often used today because of their reputation as "speed" in the 1950s and 1960s, as well as orexigenic agents to aid weight loss. Their addictive properties discouraged their use, even for legitimate needs. A congener, *methylphenidate* was supposed to be metabolized differently to minimize middosage withdrawal and was the primary stimulant used as an adjuvant analgesic. Methylphenidate itself developed a checkered reputation when identified as a treatment for attention deficit disorder with hyperactivity. It was believed that such methylphenidate became overprescribed as an antidote for overcrowded classrooms or to quiet the natural curiosity of a child in a school setting. The idiosyncratic effect of a stimulant calming or focusing a child was at odds with its known energizing or activating properties thought to stimulate brain function to synchronize a hyperactive motor system with a brain that processed only at normal speeds.

This collection of properties—adjuvant analgesic, mood elevator, and energizing drug—made stimulants optimal drugs to use in cancer symptom management, particularly in fatigue. In addition to methylphenidate, other stimulant preparations such as *dex*methylphenidate (marketed as Focalin® and others) approved for attention deficit hyperactivity in children and modafinil (Provigil® and others) approved for narcolepsy and daytime sleepiness have been used to treat cancer-induced fatigue.[54] Armodafinil, similar to modafinil (Nuvigil® and others), has a comparable profile.

Optimal dosing of stimulants during or after cancer treatment has not been established. No matter the age of the patient, one should adopt the geriatrician's mantra, "start low and go slowly." For patients without arrhythmia, mood disorder, or drug dependence in the past, best to use a test dose of 5 mg once a day for a few days, at a time when a patient wants to be most awake and alert, and at least 5 hours before bedtime. If the patient does not experience palpitations, tachycardia, or a sense of feeling jittery (unlikely at a low dose), the medication can be continued and the dosage cautiously increased to not more than 20 to 30 mg/24 hours for most patients. It is best that patients taper off rather than stop abruptly, conservatively not more than 50% of the full 24-hour dose every 3 days.

Rarely do patients use more than 10 mg/day or equivalent dose of methylphenidate on an ongoing basis. Selected patients with advanced cancers are most appreciative of the extra energy and wakefulness that the medication provides, reinforced by data from Lasheen and colleagues.[55] Because of the many potential interactions with the variety of drugs used during cancer treatment, experience tells us to avoid long-acting preparations that can leave patients who do experience jitteriness with side effects for too long. If patients feel a sudden letdown for 3 to 5 hours after a dose, that may be avoided by use of the *dextro* isomer, *d*-methylphenidate at comparable dosing schedules.[56]

Modafinil is marketed in the United States in dosages of 100 mg or 200 mg, with usual doses of 100 to 200 mg once a day. Open-label studies have not thus far supported individual claims.[57]

In general, antidepressants of any class have not been shown to be helpful in the treatment of fatigue. Patients do sometimes report a feeling of "increased energy" when using bupropion (marketed both as Wellbutrin® as an antidepressant and Zyban® to reduce nicotine cravings in smoking cessation), but this use has not been put to clinical trial. Not surprisingly, one way to simulate a nonprescription stimulant is to try *very* strong coffee to boost energy, with the usual caveats about arrhythmias and time of day applying.

▓ USE THE LEARN SYSTEM TO BRING THEORY TO THE PATIENT EASILY

The components of The LEARN System are ideally suited to provide help in making a quick differential diagnosis and initiating treatment for fatigue. Until more definitive investigation confirms more specific proinflammatory cytokines or antibodies, what we can do now is properly evaluate and optimize nutrition, rest, and activity. Normalizing the experience for the patient and family is a great relief. That is best done by acknowledging the symptom while accessing information and tools that help a patient and family from the start to work on minimizing symptoms.

11

The LEARN System Components: Resting and Sleeping Effectively Furthers Recovery ("**R**est" and Sleep)

Until the last 10 years, little attention has been paid to the changes in sleep that affect patients with cancer. There is no reason to suspect that sleep and rest are any less restorative in the recovery from cancer and treatment than they are for the health of the general population.

Sleep disorders with importance in cancer include insomnias, hypersomnias (daytime sleepiness), circadian disorders, and obstructive sleep disorders. Obstructive disorders are of particular concern for patients with head and neck cancer or lung cancer. A further overlap area of interest is in the sleep interruption from hot flashes affecting breast and prostate cancer patients. Flashes often wake patients up at night and nonhormonal drugs tested to treat hot flashes are mostly sedating, which may suppress or allow a patient to disregard nighttime flashes. It is not yet known if they are also helpful to treat general sleep problems in cancer patients.

▓ CANCER TREATMENT THAT DIRECTLY AFFECTS SLEEP

Changes in sleep patterns are common in patients with cancer, and estimates can run three times higher than in the general population.[58] That prevalence varies with type of cancer, type of treatment, age, comorbidities, type and phase of treatment, and how it is evaluated. Interrupted sleep is a symptom that deserves attention because of its effect on quality of life, and possibly a more direct effect on treatment outcome.

With much of sleep controlled centrally, and the recognition that so much of cancer treatment affects the central nervous system, the area is fertile for research and creative thought. In a surgical oncology service treating head and neck and urology patients, 78% postoperatively reported taking too long to fall asleep, nighttime wakening, and daytime napping.[59] A large study of more than 800 patients during chemotherapy for various cancers concluded that poor sleep persisted through chemotherapy, being underrecognized, undermanaged, and understudied. So many of the medications used during treatment affect the sleep–wake cycle, including around-the-clock use of opioids, daytime use of antiemetics with sedating properties, and the use of corticosteroids as antiemetics and primary treatment. Associations between interleukin-6 (IL-6) with sleep efficiency and duration were discovered during testing of a home-based exercise intervention for breast and prostate cancer patients receiving radiation therapy.[60] Those with advanced cancer also endorsed a poor quality of sleep despite "normal" duration.[61]

▩ REST/SLEEP RELATES TO OTHER PROMINENT SYMPTOMS

Because of the difficulty in assessing sleep as a symptom in isolation, it is logical to con-clude that sleep duration and quality affect levels of fatigue, mood, and pain, and that their successful management requires some coordination of activity, rest, optimal nutri-tion, and education. Where office assessment is most likely done as part of an interval history during follow-up visits, researchers use tailored questionnaires, items in symp-tom management, or distress assessments. More specific physiologic correlates are mea-sured by movement with an actigraphic device or more sophisticated polysomnography, assessing brain electrical activity, eye and jaw muscle movement, leg muscle movement, airflow, respiratory effort, electrocardiogram (EKG), and oxygen saturation.

Efforts to prevent sleep difficulties that preexist cancer have been suggested. Berger and colleagues tested a behavioral-cognitive intervention before chemotherapy and reinforced it during treatment.[62]

▩ CANCER-SPECIFIC TREATMENT OF SLEEP DISORDERS

Despite the robust direct-to-consumer marketing campaigns in the media, it is unclear if sedative–hypnotic medications should be the first line treatments for insomnia, or if they are used, should be prescribed for short time and combined with environmental changes. In noncancer populations, ramelteon (Rozerem®), a melatonin receptor agonist is a new approach to insomnia that does not carry tolerance or dependence. The product works best to help someone fall asleep, not stay asleep. Being such a newly licensed drug, it may be too soon to see reports after more widespread use. Ramelteon has not been tested in cancer patients, and should be considered with caution because changing circadian rhythms and melatonin-like substances may potentiate or interfere with treatments.[63,64]

The often necessary daytime use of opioids, benzodiazepine antiemetics (such as lora-zepam or Ativan® and others), phenothiazine/benzamide antiemetics (prochlorperazine or Compazine® and others; metoclopramide or Reglan® and others), and diphenhy-dramine (Benadryl® and others) almost uniformly cause daytime sedation, affecting the sleep–wake cycle. Using sedating medications during the day changes how we fall asleep and stay asleep at night. It may be unrealistic to expect a *usual* night's sleep, even if some accommodation is made for being off one's regular schedule and expected cancer-related distress. As with the treatment of other symptoms, knowing what has been found effica-cious in a noncancer population and tailoring those findings to the special circumstances of patients with cancer will be the most helpful, short of controlled trials.

In other special populations who are at risk for chronic insomnia, strategies have been developed to avoid the potential long-term side effects of benzodiazepines, such as falls and drug-related daytime memory impairment. One strategy is the off-label use of sedating medications such as trazodone (Desyrel®) or tricyclic antidepressants. Trazodone use in men runs a small risk of priapism, but otherwise is well tolerated for sleep (50-100 mg hs) for both genders at doses lower than used for depression. Tricyclic antidepressants have been long used in oncology as a primary treatment for neuropathic pain, but their anticholinergic side effects augment constipation and dryness from opioids and antiemetics. Doses of nortriptyline 10-50 mg hs, or doxepin 25-50 mg hs are quite sedating without any risk of tolerance or dependence, but similarly drying. For patients with chemotherapy-related neuropathy or diarrhea from pelvic radiotherapy or 5-fluorouracil, the troublesome secondary effects may actually be beneficial to certain subgroups in which one drug can treat two symptoms.

Newer generations of antidepressants have also been used for sleep and sedation as an alternative to benzodiazepines. Short of trials using improvement in mood as a primary outcome, the sedating properties of serotonin reuptake inhibitors (paroxetine or Paxil® and others, sertraline or Zoloft® and others) have been used quite extensively to suppress hot flashes in patients with androgen or estrogen suppression and are of particular help in minimizing waking at night. This helpful nighttime effect has drawn colleagues to prescribe antidepressants off-label as sleep aids. Concerns over certain cytochrome P450 interactions in patients on tamoxifen have heightened our awareness to the myriad of potential P450 interactions. Some pharmacy databases or larger cancer centers in which pharmacists do rounds with clinical teams can be helpful to triage for patients whose drug combinations may put them at risk for interactions. Serotonin-norepinepherine reuptake inhibitors such as venlafaxine (Effexor and others) are minimally metabolized at a cytochrome P450 2D6 locus, and may be an alternative to other serotonin reuptake inhibitors.[65]

Alternative supplements or substances do not offer preferable alternatives thus far. The relationship between altered circadian rhythms and the development of cancer has been dubious, so advising over-the-counter melatonin supplementation or ramelteon is questionable. The popularized notion that the amino acid tryptophan can be used as a sedative was born out of our perceived tiredness after significant turkey consumption containing dietary tryptophan, often at a Thanksgiving meal. The safety of concentrated tryptophan supplements has come under scrutiny because of its hepatotoxicity. Other sedating supplements such as valerian and kava kava have been associated with safety concerns that discourage their use. Although alcoholic beverages are often relaxing and sedating, such an effect is short-lived, and the resulting rebound stimulation as the alcohol wears off disrupts sleep rather than enhance it. Because alcohol promotes certain cancers and because of a variety of other dangers, common sense tells us to discourage usage beyond a minimal amount.

▓ NONPHARMACOLOGIC APPROACHES

Perhaps the most attractive approaches to improving sleep during cancer treatment are not drug related. What is often described in shorthand as *cognitive behavioral therapies* is largely a specialized educational intervention that

- provides information about how we fall and stay asleep
- focuses on how to adjust the environment and presleep activities to promote good quality and length of sleep
  - using the bedroom for sleep and sex
  - cooling the room temperature

- limiting caffeine to early in day
- avoiding exercise, heavy meals, or stimulating activities at bedtime such as answering e-mail
- using silicone earplugs to block out ambient noise or sleep partner's snoring
- wearing eye masks
- having opaque window treatments that block outside light (street lamps)
- using white noise or wave sound machines to block ambient noise and focus on a bland sound
- cooling a room by lowering heat or cracking open a window
- taking a warm (not scalding hot) bath to cool the body afterward at bedtime
- placing electronic devices on silent and out of reach
• schedules consistent periods of sleep and wakefulness every day of the week
• uses distraction: quiet reading or soothing music
• uses massage to relax skeletal muscle
• introduces progressive muscle relaxation training

Virtually, side-effect free, these tips can supply patients and families with things they can do if you are unable to access specialized sleep counseling for cancer patients in which you practice.

▣ THE CONCEPT OF *REST*: DOES IT EXTEND THE BENEFITS OF SLEEP?

Because of the inevitability of the use of sedating opioids and antiemetics that cannot be avoided postoperatively, during radiation therapy or chemotherapy, the use of day-time periods of rest may further interrupt nighttime sleep, but provide a patient with the time needed for recovery tailored to the rhythms of cancer treatment.

As the clinical implications of sleep have only recently come under scientific scrutiny, activities that encompass *rest* are even less investigated. With the absence of pharmacologic interest in promoting rest, it is unlikely that techniques for more effective resting will be put to clinical trial. In keeping with the concept of proposing potentially helpful treatment that has few to no toxicities, finite periods of rest can be "prescribed" in good conscience and responsibly.

Suggestions about how to encourage rest overlap significantly with those that promote sleep with some additional suggestions to be entertained. Individual variation and preference make one activity restful to some and not others. Noise-blocking earplugs or electronic noise-canceling earphones can help block out ambient noise. High volume music listened to through earbuds can be restful to some and distasteful to others (putting aside the ill effects of loud music on hearing loss). Activities that distract are similarly acceptable to different people, and what may be acceptable at the start of treatment may become irritating with progressive disease, as the time of being sick passes. Commonly suggested ways to promote rest include—but are certainly not limited to—music, reading, repetitive tasks, and time spent with one's own pet or one from a community agency offering animal assisted visits. A study looking at the efficacy of animal assisted visits on patients receiving combined chemotherapy and radiation therapy is underway—funded by the Good Dog Foundation and Pfizer Animal Health. Measured outcomes are quality of life, amount of analgesics and antiemetics used, and adherence to treatment schedules.*

Recent interest in *relaxation training* and *yoga* are efforts to encourage activities promoting rest. Nomenclature becomes somewhat varied. The techniques in progressive muscle relaxation overlap with those taught in *self-hypnosis*, which is misunderstood by the public because of its popularization in entertainment. Hypnosis in some circles is considered a medical therapy, which entails certification and scope of practice for some professionals in some states or cancer centers. Yoga's association with its spiritual roots in Eastern philosophy made its standing dubious in cancer centers, but has now moved into the mainstream as a modality that promotes rest, flexibility, and resistance training. How we think about or categorize activities like relaxation training or yoga becomes important. Some patients are uncomfortable with its inclusion as a *complementary* or *alternative* treatment. Some clinicians are concerned about the implications that its practice can help prevent cancer may get confused with its helpful effects as an adjunct to optimal care. For others, its aura as a modality outside of the mainstream makes it more attractive for them to learn and use.

The American Cancer Society lists acupuncture, aromatherapy, art therapy, biofeedback, labyrinth walking, massage therapy, meditation, music therapy, prayer and spirituality, tai chi, and yoga as "complimentary approaches that may be used with cancer treatment."[66] Putting aside politics and spirituality, these activities promote relaxation, diversion, and some modality as a common thread. Although some have been put to clinical trials, each has negligible to minimal risk of side effects. And apart from isolated and rare untoward effects (such as cellulites from acupuncture needle insertion), they are considered safe ways to foster relaxation or diversion in various ways, with additional potential benefits through each modality (music therapy or art therapy).

Gilda's Club has taken a step further to bring these and other modalities to patients and families through its worldwide centers and programming. Through lectures, workshops, and innovations like Noogieland with special kids programs that foster play and social support, such services are available in many locales. *Noogieland* offers mutual support for kids with cancer and those who are family members of someone with cancer, using art, distraction, and camaraderie. The program also offers respite for the adult patient an extra opportunity to catch up on their rest.

▥ USE THE LEARN SYSTEM TO BRING THEORY TO THE PATIENT EASILY

The oncology subspecialist is often the first provider to manage sleep problems since the culture of insomnia, fueled by direct-to-consumer marketing, makes us turn to prescription drugs for relief first. With the prevalence of the use of lorazepam as an

---

* Continuing in the spirit of full disclosure, I am the principal investigator of the study.

The
LEARN
System©

p. 141
My Weekly
Recovery
Planner

antiemetic, patients already have a benzodiazepine in their medication chest. With the advances in sleep medicine over recent years and the latest interest in sleep during cancer treatment, the imperative to pass on this information in the midst of a busy practice is simplified by using The LEARN System, which summarizes the importance of using nonpharmacologic approaches, in advance of or in addition to sedative-hypnotics. The clinicians' endorsement and even promotion of the information is vital for patients and families to accept it and use the system. Patients and families will be able to see their progress when reviewing *My Weekly Recovery Planner*, and bring the information you need to quickly evaluate and see which prescriptions are necessary.

Clinicians may wonder why prescribing rest is necessary at all. Many, but not all, patients do admit that they feel a certain time pressure to do as much as they can while they can after being diagnosed with a life-threatening illness. Candidly, patients will discuss how, out of fear, that they (or their families and workplaces) will miss them and their contributions, and they will miss being there, so they try to "pack in" as much as possible at a time when fatigue stands in their way. Being advised to use short periods of rest effectively is very helpful. Patients at the very end of life may have the desire, but not the energy reserves to exceed their abilities.

12

The LEARN System Components: Maintaining Optimal Nutrition Eases Time in Treatment and Recovery ("Nutrition")

Weight changes that occur because of cancer or its treatment are common. Although weight loss is commonly described, weight gain is an important symptom requiring specific management for a subgroup of patients, many of whom have hormonally dependent prostate or breast cancer. Both weight loss and weight gain adversely affect morbidity and mortality, with 80% of patients risking life-threatening consequences from cancer cachexia.[67] The widespread effect of weight change in cancer patients is owed in part to the decreased resistance to infection and effect on thrombosis. When even an intuitive grandmother recognizes that "you don't die of cancer, you die from something else," such an observation underscores the importance of nutritional changes from cancer.

▦ WEIGHT LOSS

Weight loss in cancer means more than just not wanting to eat. Before pathophysiological mechanisms could be identified, it was common to believe that "if (s)he just ate a little more," the weight loss could be reversed. We know today that the mechanism of weight loss is not as simple as that, and providing a few calories alone does not reverse the symptom.

Weight loss occurs with a variety of other comorbidities. Chronic conditions that lead to weight loss include kidney or liver failure, chronic obstructive pulmonary disease (COPD), or heart failure. Acutely ill patients with sepsis, trauma, or burns also lose weight quickly. Caloric supplementation will help counteract weight loss in these acute situations. Weight loss in HIV disease often occurs with refractory disease, with weight gain as a common side effect of some current antiretroviral regimens.

In cancer, it is helpful to think about the factors causing weight loss in two categories: those *associated* with weight loss and those that actually *induce* cancer weight loss.

Cancer-*Associated* Weight Loss	Cancer-*Induced* Weight Loss
Obstruction	Metabolic changes
Treatment side effects	Inflammatory cytokines
Practical causes	*No weight gain* with additional protein
Adding proteins and energy source *may* help gain weight	and energy sources

Cancer-Associated Weight Loss

A useful way to summarize those factors involved with cancer-associated weight loss is to start at the top of the head and work down to the lower extremities: general fatigue and deconditioning; worry; isolation and depression; changes in smell, taste, or sight of food; motor control of swallowing; inability to sustain energy to chew and swallow; xerostomia; mucositis or stomatitis; obstruction; esophagitis; gastroparesis; gastrointestinal side effects of chemotherapy; corticosteroids or systemic antibiotics; secondary colitis; presence of colostomies or urostomies; constipation induced by a host of medications used in cancer treatment; diarrhea associated with pelvic radiation; lymphedema; peripheral neuropathy; and generalized weakness hindering shopping, cooking, and cleaning up.

Cancer-associated weight loss can often be ameliorated by direct correction of the symptoms when possible as well as by augmenting calorie-rich proteins and sources of energy to boost intake through the oral or parenteral routes, as in non-cancer acute conditions.

Patients with cancer-associated weight loss can greatly benefit from nutritional counseling from an experienced registered dietician or nutritionist. Adapting food preferences to add calories that are rich in proteins and complex carbohydrates needs personalized advice. Patients and caregivers are often reluctant to use parenteral feedings through a percutaneous endoscopic gastrostomy (PEG) or percutaneous endoscopic jejunostomy (PEJ) in fear that once inserted the tube, it will be permanent. The use of total parenteral nutrition (TPN) or peripheral parenteral nutrition (PPN) can be quite helpful for selected patients with a specific goal in mind, such as preoperatively or part of critical care. Specialized formulas that can be used orally or parenterally remain the mainstay of intervention with this group. See the Worksheets.

Cancer-Induced Weight Loss

The more challenging aspect of weight loss in cancer is the understanding and treatment of cancer-induced weight loss. This is often referred to as the cancer cachexia syndrome. The term *cachexia* derived from the Greek (κακοV ηξιV) meaning "a bad condition" is a complex condition that involves wasting, fatigue, early satiety, and sensory changes.[68] Because the condition is often mislabeled as *anorexia–cachexia*, inclusion of the term anorexia can lead to an improper conclusion that there is a relationship to anorexia nervosa. Cancer-induced weight loss has much less, if any, psychological component; patients and colleagues should not be led to the erroneous conclusion that there is more voluntary control over the condition than exists.

Lasheen and Walsh[69] identified specific symptoms of cancer-induced weight loss: early satiety, constipation, nausea, taste changes, vomiting, dysphagia, fatigue, weakness, and lack of energy. Inherent in the process is the loss of skeletal muscle with or without fat[70] associated with appetite loss, inflammation, and insulin resistance. Increased lipolysis through an increased expression of hormone sensitive lipase has been

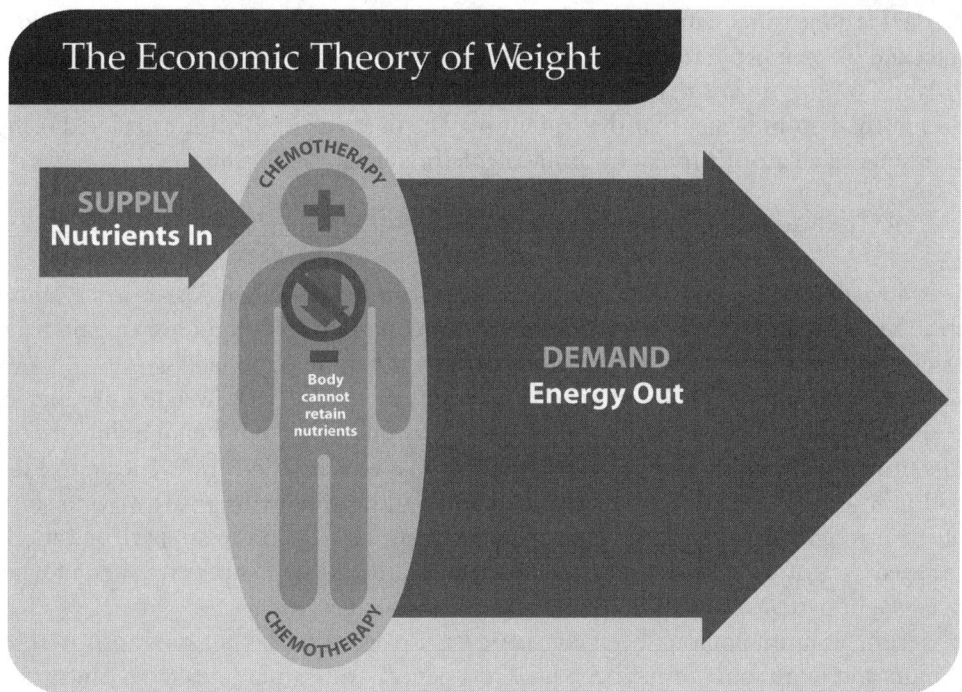

Obstacles to maintaining weight: The energy demands on the body during chemotherapy far exceed the amount of calories a person can comfortably consume in a day. Plus, chemotherapy can inhibit the body's ability to retain some nutrients.

identified in animal models. In vivo, the role of proinflammatory and inflammatory cytokines is intimately involved in the process, with a direct destruction of skeletal muscle, all contributing to the perception that a patient's appearance is described as *skin and bones.*

Once observed only as a part of progressive cancer illness, more subtle forms of cachexia are receiving greater attention earlier in the course of cancer with the goal of preventing the weight loss and metabolic breakdown.[71]

As an educational tool, weight maintenance can be understood as a model of economics: balancing assets, expenses, and savings. *Learn to Live Through Cancer: What You Need to Know and Do* features this graphic as a comparison to a model of personal finance familiar to mostly everyone.

Specific assessment tools that are valid and reliable are under development or being tested to identify patients at risk for weight loss. The Mini-Nutritional Assessment has been used by Gioulbasanis and colleagues[72] and has been found to be more predictive than asking about weight loss alone. Gabison and colleagues[73] showed the Cachexia Assessment Scale to be both valid and reliable as well. Body mass index (BMI) is routinely used outside of cancer treatment to differentiate between individuals who are underweight, normal weight, overweight, or obese, and can easily be used in the office setting as a triage tool for cachexia, although it is not a predictor of short- or long-term outcome in specific cancers such as esophageal.[74]

BMI is a measurement of body fat based on height and weight that applies to both men and women between the ages of 18 and 65 years. A healthy BMI score is between 20 and 25. A score less than 20 indicates that a patient may be underweight; a value greater than 25 indicates that the patient may be overweight. BMI is calculated using an online calculator (http://www.bmi-calculator.net) or the formula:

$$BMI = (\text{weight in pounds}) / (\text{height in inches} \times \text{height in inches}) \times 703$$

A low normal or low BMI often precedes significant weight loss during cancer treatment. Tracking BMIs as well as documenting patterns of weight loss or gain prior to diagnosis comprise basic information used by nutritional specialists.

Loss of weight is usually expressed as a percentage of body weight (number of pounds lost / baseline weight in pounds). It is generally accepted that an unintentional loss in body weight greater than 10% during cancer is a serious threat to morbidity and mortality. Such a simple calculation can be misleading with a patient who starts out overweight or obese. The loss of skeletal muscle, a prominent part of cancer-induced weight loss, remains as much of a hazard during cancer treatment for an overweight patient, so the threshold for concern is equal.

Serum albumin has long been considered a surrogate marker for prognosis in solid tumors and lymphoma. It has been used as a general indicator of health in cancer and as a predictor of poor outcome.[75]

Imaging has not traditionally been helpful in the evaluation of cancer-induced weight loss. Prado and colleagues[76] reported on the potential use of computerized tomography (CT) scans to quantify relative amounts of lean and adipose body tissues as an aid to understanding cancer cachexia.

A prudent signal for nutritional intervention should be a loss of 5% of body weight without regard to initial BMI so that patients can maximize their quality of life, reduce the morbidities of treatment, and maximize treatment response. A patient's weight in comparison to his or her gender-specific *ideal body weight* (*IBW*) can corroborate the need for nutritional intervention.

Mechanisms of Cancer Cachexia and Cancer-Induced Weight Loss

With the recognition of the widespread effects of proinflammatory cytokines in cancer, much has been identified that contributes to understanding the mechanism of cancer-induced cachexia. Expanding on the long-held models of cancer growth, it is now well established that apart from local extension, hematogenous spread, and lymphatic involvement, cytokines mediate the effects of cancer on multiple end organs. Meta-analyses have identified over 80 studies that have evaluated the role of systemic inflammatory responses using biochemical or hematological markers,[77] although their use in assessment is not advised outside of a clinical trial.

Hormonal influences via leptin[78] and ghrelin have also been related to the changes in weight and body composition in cancer-induced weight loss through their influence on satiety. Ghrelin, which is predominantly secreted by gastric endocrine cells, stimulates food intake and triggers a positive energy balance through a central mechanism involving hypothalamic neuropeptides.[79]

■ CYTOKINES INCREASE THE METABOLIC ACTIVITY OF CELLS THAT EXPEND CALORIES

The mechanisms of cancer-induced weight loss underscore the interference of cell-mediated inflammatory cytokines in the maintenance of weight during treatment for cancer. Cachectin (tumor necrosis factor alpha [TNF-α]), interleukins-1 and -6, and C-reactive protein have an imputed role in the inability to retain protein stored as lean body mass for energy and well-being. In the schematic, the circulating cytokines enter the cell and encourage metabolic activity of cancer cells, raising the energy requirements even more. Glucose serves as an energy supply for only a few hours after it is consumed and digested. Extra calories are stored as glycogen, providing another few hours of energy supply. After these initial glycogen stores are depleted, extraction

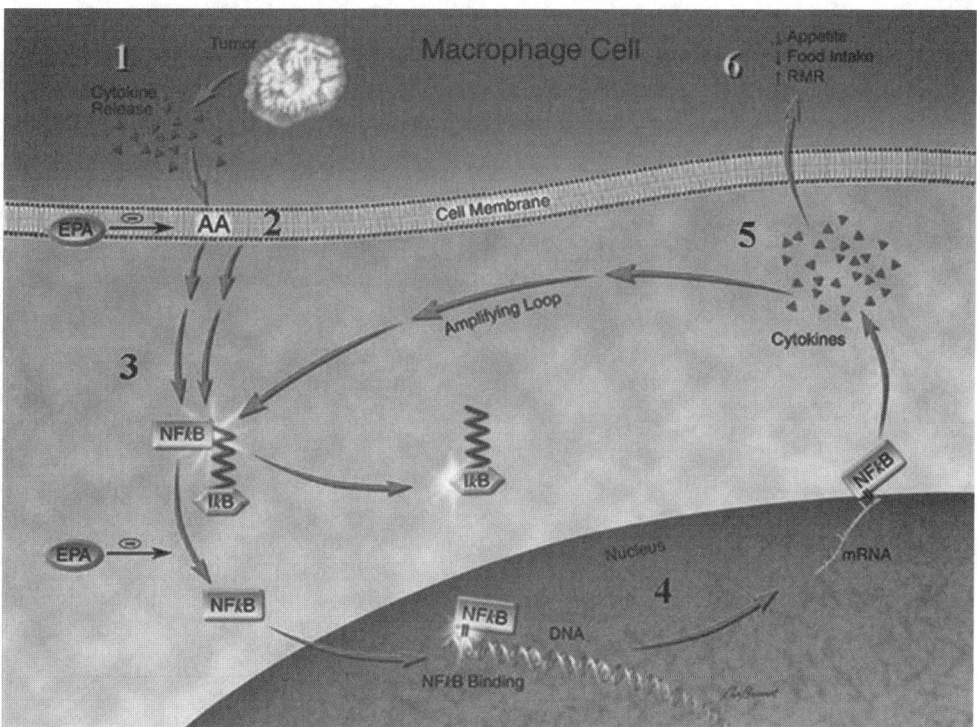

Slide 12.1 This illustration shows graphically how a cancer cell goes into *overdrive*. The large cancer cell absorbs the *cytokine* unless the EPA (eicosapentonic acid, an important omega-3 fatty acid fish oil) binds the *AA* (*arachadonic acid*) in the cell wall. If the cytokine enters, then the cell soaks up calories in overdrive. Copyright Abbott Laboratories. Reprinted with permission.

of energy from fat cells uses too many calories, so proteins stored as lean body mass are accessed.

It has also been proposed that the proinflammatory cytokines act on the central nervous system as well to alter the release and function of several neurotransmitters, affecting both appetite and metabolic rate.[80]

CYTOKINES ENCOURAGE SKELETAL MUSCLE WASTING

An additional cytokine, proteolysis-inducing factor (PIF), further fuels the use of lean body mass for energy (depleting muscles and worsening fatigue) and aggravating cachexia even more. Support of the resting energy expenditure—the amount of energy the body needs for minimal sustenance—is mediated through the same cytokines, which use further calories because tissues demand energy. Dodson and colleagues[81] associate this phenomenon with wasting, anemia, reduced caloric intake,

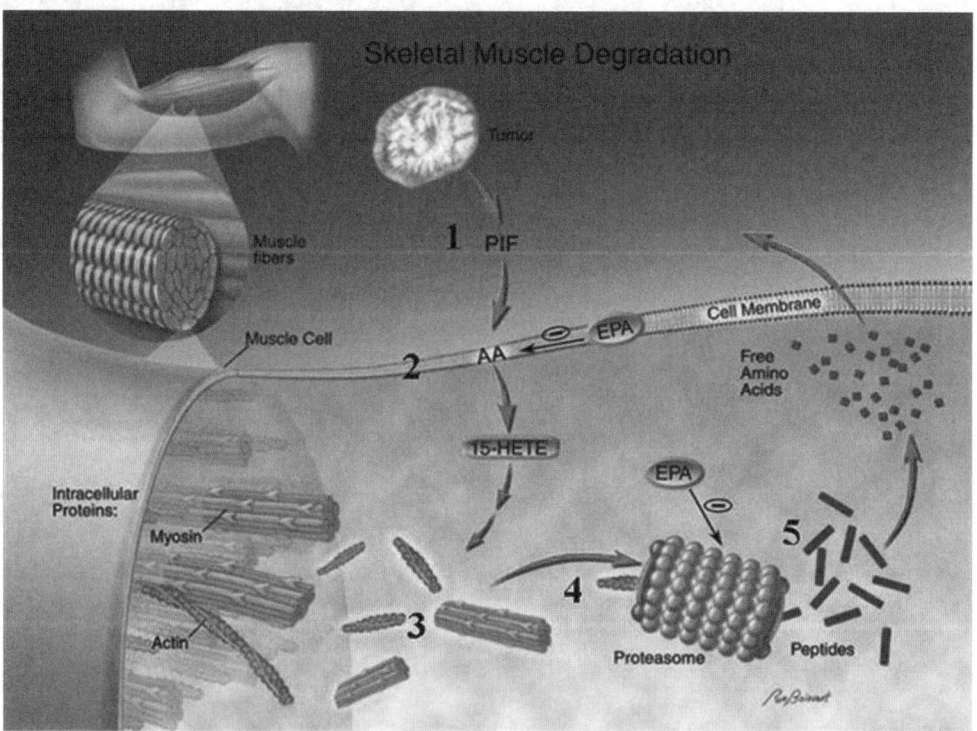

Slide 12.2 Cytokines will similarly enter skeletal muscle, increasing its need for calories, causing weight loss unless opposed by the EPA fish oils that bind the AA so that the cytokines cannot enter the muscle cells. Copyright Abbott Laboratories. Reprinted with permission.

altered immune function, increased disability, fatigue, diminished quality of life, and reduced survival.

VITAMIN SUPPLEMENTATION

Whether caused by an ever-growing supplement industry or the desire to improve our nutrition with a pill, much information—good and bad—alleges the use of vitamin supplements as a way to "protect" healthy tissues from the cytotoxic effects of chemo-therapy and radiation therapy. Patients often think about taking vitamin supplements purported to reduce cancer risk *after* diagnosis in an effort to keep them healthy. It is generally accepted that a usual physiological dose of multivitamin can be safely taken during treatment, and that to avoid making treatments less effective, higher doses of vitamins A, C, and E are best left after treatment is completed.[82] New interest in the supplementation of vitamin D[83] in breast and prostate cancers may change guidelines in the future.

INTERVENTIONS

Adequate Intake Alone, Insufficient But Necessary

Effective interventions to overcome weight loss in cancer also address three economic components: supply, energy, and demand. Provision of adequate proteins, high-quality complex carbohydrates, and lipids are the cornerstone to overcome *supply* deficits. Nutritional counseling and the use of personalized meal plans or fortified, specially pre-pared foods that can be swallowed or administered via PEG or PEJ are tailor-made to an individual's comorbidities, including diabetes or protein intolerance, such as sprue. Com-mercially made food supplements can be used orally or parenterally, although some trial and error may be necessary to find a brand or product easily tolerated. Insurance reim-bursement identifying preferred products based on contractual agreements may also dic-tate which supplement is used. When using parenteral supplements, small regular feeds through a plunger or overnight feeds via pump allow for the adequate caloric intake.

The dietary patterns in patients with advanced cancer are not well known. In a study on 151 patients, a wide variation in the intake of energy and protein was observed.[84] Even the subjects with highest intake had a recent history of weight loss, suggesting that diets of even those people were consistently inadequate for weight maintenance. Cluster analysis found three dietary patterns that differed in food choice and caloric intake: (1) the milk and soup pattern; (2) the fruit and white bread pattern; and (3) the meat and potato pattern of intake. Low intakes and high risk of weight loss were associated with decreased frequency of eating, and the subjects' dietary profiles included little variety and had unusually high proportions of liquids. It was postulated that a doubling or even tripling of dietary intake would be necessary to maintain weight. This is an unrealistic goal when patients are suffering from cachexia.

■ MAXIMIZING THE RETENTION OF CALORIES AS AN ENERGY SOURCE

Pharmacologic stimulation of appetite by corticosteroids, megestrol acetate, or dronabinol and nabilone (cannabis congeners) can each encourage maintenance or additional intake (see Table 12.1). It has been demonstrated that one of the possible mechanisms that antagonize the progression of cachexia lies in the endocannabinoid system. Cannabinoid type 1 receptor activation is shown to stimulate appetite-promoting lipogenesis and energy storage.[85] Further development of safe cannabinoids may help reduce cancer patient's cachectic state. Cyproheptadine, a seratonergic antihistamine, has been used despite its sedative properties. Prokinetic agents such as metoclopramide may help with feelings of early satiety or when PEG feedings leave one feeling "full," even though small quantities have been instilled. Omega-3 fatty acids containing eicosapentaenoic acid (EPA) and docosahexaenoic acid (DHA) are thought to downregulate the cytokines to help maintain lean body mass and minimize the use of proteins as an energy source to augment energy retention. As a food supplement rather than a prescription drug item, omega-3s have been overlooked as a mainstay in the treatment of cancer cachexia. The substance has been tested alone and in conjunction with high protein and carbohydrate food supplements, and is currently marketed outside the United States for cancer cachexia.

Studies in pancreatic cancer,[86] head and neck cancer,[87] and lung cancer[88] have shown merit in omega-3s' effectiveness in the retention of lean body mass, and the optimal component of weight gain at approximately 2,000 mg/day. Although omega-3 fatty acid esters are Food and Drug Administration (FDA)-approved as a prescription drug for hypertriglyceridemia (Lovaza®; formerly Omacor®), they can be recommended as an *off-label* indication in the United States. The purported mechanism of EPA and DHA is illustrated in Slide 12.1. EPA is shown binding to AA, arachidonic acid in the cell wall, blocking the passage of the destructive cytokines into the cell, reducing the inflated caloric needs and preserving weight.

In the Bruera and colleagues' 2003 trial,[85] EPA has been compared to placebo. The patients were randomized to receive 180 mg EPA, 120 mg DHA, and 1 mg vitamin E or placebo. In this trial, the patients were not able to tolerate 18 capsules per day. The comparison of results showed a slight weight gain with EPA, DHA, and vitamin E. Another study compared different doses of EPA alone and megestrol acetate alone to combinations of EPA.[89] The combination of EPA with megestrol acetate resulted in a worse outcome versus megestrol acetate alone. The benefits of weight gain showed no significant difference between EPA alone and megestrol alone. Antilipolytic treatment is shown to prevent cachexia progression.

Lundholm and colleagues[90] evaluated whether daily, long-acting insulin attenuates the progression of weight loss in cancer patients without any harmful side effects. Criteria used for measuring results were nutritional assessment, blood tests, indirect calorimetry, maximum exercise test, quality of life, and daily physical activity. The results showed body fat in the trunk and legs was significantly higher among the patients receiving insulin compared to controls. Insulin improved the metabolic efficiency during exercise, ultimately leading to the conclusion that

TABLE 12.1 Pharmacologic Stimulation of Appetite or Weight Gain

Class of Agent	Name	Effects	Side Effects
Glucocorticoids	methylprednisolone dexamethasone Prednisone® Decadron®	↓ nausea, antiemetic transient ↑ appetite *no* effect on lean body mass	jittery → agitation insomnia, mood swings gastritis, reflux weaken proximal muscles (to stand from prone or seated position) avascular necrosis of the hips (protracted course)
Anabolic steroids	oxandrolone (Oxandrin®)	↑ lean body mass & weight	agitation, hepatic insufficiency, acne, edema
Progestational agents megestrol acetate	(Megace®)	increase appetite *no* effect on lean body mass	risk of blood clots (thrombosis) surprising lack of feminizing side effects
Cannabinoids	dronabinol (Marinol®), nabilone (Cesamet®)	↓ nausea, antiemetic "munchies"	"stoned," "high"
Antiserotoninergic antihistamine	cyproheptadine (Periactin®)	minimal weight gain	drowsiness, sedation
Neuroleptics	olanzapine (Zyprexa®)	increased weight	relative hyperglycemia may be responsible for weight gain can lead to type II diabetes
Omega-3 fatty acids	omega-3 esters (Lovaza® or Omacor®)	increased lean body mass	underused due to stigma as a nonprescription food supplement
Thalidomide	Thalomid®	decreased weight loss	some sedation; must use effective barrier contraception to avoid teratogenic effects

insulin is a significant metabolic treatment in the multimodal palliation of weight loss in cancer patients.[91,92]

Essential amino acids such as arginine, glutamine, and hydroxymethylbutyric acid (HMB) further inhibit PIF to maintain lean body mass. Commercial preparations containing amino-acid rich supplements (Juven® and others) have also been used for the frail elderly without cancer to promote wound healing. These essential amino acids are also marketed separately as food supplements. An early attempt to prove the efficacy of another supplement, hydrazine sulfate, failed to show it as an effective substance in cancer cachexia in patients with advanced lung or colorectal cancer.[93]

APPETITE STIMULATION

Appetite stimulation alone often has providers and families believe that *something* is being done to reverse or avoid weight loss, but such efforts do not result in weight stabilization or weight gain. The effects of corticosteroids are transient at best and often result in steroid myopathy with proximal muscle weakness, infection, or gastritis. They are often confused with anabolic steroids when suggested in the context of weight gain or weight maintenance, and patients and families are unduly worried about "'roid rage" as a potential side effect. Prescription anabolic steroids (oxandrolone [Oxandrin®]) and others when monitored closely can be of great help in selected patients.

Cannabinoids (dronabinol [Marinol®] and nabilone [Cesamet®]) can increase appetite, particularly the urge to snack, as can smoked marijuana when without risk of contaminants or legal concerns. Megestrol acetate (Megace® and others) effectively add water and fat to show weight gain. Older clinicians who used it as an antiestrogen treatment before selective estrogen receptor blockers are comfortable using it as a first line at a dosage of 600 to 800 mg/day in a concentrated liquid preparation.

MULTIDISCIPLINARY MANAGEMENT IS OPTIMAL

An example of how the multidisciplinary team can work at its best is in the evaluation and treatment of cancer cachexia. Often, the initial evaluation is made by the oncology subspecialists or oncology nurses who note the falling weight and loss of lean body mass and are in the best position to make (and seek insurance authorization for, when possible) referral to a dietician or oncology nutritionist who assesses the patient for food preferences and adapts those to maintaining weight or reversing weight loss. Matching the proper product or homemade recipe for calorie supplementation is often best done by the dietician or nutritionist. Parenteral feeds via PEG or PEJ must involve the dietician for teaching and ongoing monitoring. The oncology nutritionist or dietician works with the social worker to access insurance benefits or entitlements, to counsel the family to help as early as possible, and to make food available rather than force it on the patient. Coordination with physical or occupational therapist can evaluate and suggest activities that can encourage appetite as well as reduce fatigue. Prescription appetite stimulants can be vetted and provided by a nurse practitioner or oncologist in concert with the other providers.[94,95]

A reasonable proactive approach is to refer all patients with cancers in which weight loss is likely to occur *early* in the course of care, so that the weight loss can be prevented, if possible. Patients with lung, pancreatic, and other gastrointestinal cancers and head and neck cancer should see the dietician or oncology nutritionist at the beginning of their treatment. In the absence of uniform guidelines for nutritional services, the clinician should review weight history (highest and lowest weights and their circumstances), food preferences, BMI, ideal body weight, as well as recommended interventions to avoid weight loss. Those would include use and choice of commercially prepared supplements, homemade foods to supply the proper number of calories from varied sources, successful strategies for weight maintenance, training for PEG or PEJ (if to be placed), triage for TPN or PPN (if indicated), and a monitoring plan.

To date, reimbursement for nutritional services in cancer is spotty. Medicare covers the services of a certified registered dietician if a patient has a comorbidity of end-stage renal disease or diabetes mellitus. Private insurance carriers may or may not elect to reimburse nutritional services. Physician services for the evaluation and management of cancer cachexia vary geographically if local codes supersede those of Medicare. Medicaid programs vary in coverage as well. Many insurance plans, under durable medical equipment or through pharmacy benefits, cover commercially prepared supplements, with some covering *only those used parenterally*. Some do not cover supplements at all to avoid offsetting home food budgets with medical reimbursement.

Traditionally, regardless of culture or tradition, food symbolizes basic sustenance, respect, celebration, socialization, and/or diversion. Woven into the fabric of daily life and ritual, when food is connected to medical treatment, decision making takes on additional layers of complexity. For example, in the health professions, we know that withholding food evolves into a moral, ethical, and religious issue that overarches society and medicine. The emblematic significance of food as succor—for patients as well as their caregivers—cannot be disregarded or taken lightly. Consider the poignant scene often played out at home or in a tertiary care cancer center: A well-meaning and frightened family member bends over at a loved one's bedside, slowly feeding scant milliliters of soup or dairy product right after the patient's episode of vomiting or as the patient is at end of life. This all-too-frequent tender gesture represents the belief that maintaining nutrition maintains the patient's life force. With so much of modern cancer treatment, a passive experience for a patient and family, feeding translates into an opportunity to "do something" active and participatory. Such noble efforts must, of course, be weighed against the risk of aspiration in the seriously ill who may actually crave the taste and texture of a familiar food as well as appreciate the human kindness and interaction. Unfortunately, such feedings add too few calories to change the course of the weight loss itself despite its secondary benefits. The psychosocial dimension of the caretaker's behavior can be seen as an *anticipatory bereavement* and is best identified by a counselor who can help the treatment team as a whole to recognize the changing goals of care.

With the loss of weight and/or appetite, a hallmark sign and symptom of major depression, behavioral health specialists in cancer must be able to ascribe it to cancer itself, the treatment, or major depression. Although yet to be shown as psychometrically valid, looking at the cause of the symptom can help make a differential diagnosis between cachexia and depression. A differentiation is often made: The *lack of motivation to eat* though able is often associated with *depression*, and the *lack of the ability to eat sufficiently* is more associated with the *cancer itself* or its treatment. Patients with significant weight loss can often smile and show a sparkle in their eyes when asked about their "favorite foods," a practical question when distinguishing between weight loss secondary to cancer cachexia or major depression.

Most religious and legal belief systems contend that nutrition and hydration are essential individual rights, and virtually every culture sees the provision of food as a basic entitlement. Optimal nutrition during initial treatment or with progressive disease is yet to be defined, but basic clinical principles and research have yielded useful techniques for the present generation of patients.

■ WEIGHT GAIN

The concern about excessive weight gain in cancer has gotten little attention until recently. With the extended survival of patients with hormone-dependent breast and prostate cancers, the interplay between weight, incidence of these cancers, survival, and quality of life are a subject of inquiry. There continues to be debate about the contribution of excess weight, particularly body fat, on the development of these cancers or the rate of recurrence after initial treatment. Excess body fat also affects the cardiac risk profile, with a shortened life span because of the development of heart disease rather than cancer progression. There are few known advantages of weight gain after cancer treatment, although anecdotally, it has been assumed that fracture rates after falls occur less often in the overweight, but that advantage may be nullified by loss of bone mineral density in patients who have received hormone suppression.

Weight and weight gain were associated with higher rates of breast cancer recurrence and mortality, most apparent in women who never smoked.[96] Androgen deprivation in men with prostate cancer has linked to a decrease in lean muscle mass, increased fat, weight gain, increased cholesterol and triglycerides, insulin resistance, loss of bone mineral density, and increased diabetes with insulin resistance.[97]

Keeping these patterns in mind, targeting both breast and prostate cancer patients at the very start of treatment is ideal. Proactive consultation with a registered dietician or oncology nutritionist is most sensible, with similar coordination with physical therapy or physical medicine and rehabilitation. Dietary guidelines particularly regarding suggestions for healthier *comfort foods* to eat during treatment that causes less weight gain is important. A more aggressive approach to this subset of patients with a long survival period is crucial.

■ USE THE LEARN SYSTEM TO BRING THEORY TO THE PATIENT EASILY

Unless your practice is at a large cancer center, it is unlikely to have an in-house registered dietician familiar with cancer. Patients will tell you, if you ask, about clinicians in the community or close-by. The oncologists' endorsement of the importance of weight management throughout the course of treatment is invaluable. Making information available to your patients and their families via up-to-date information in the public arena is a good next step. Using the tools from The LEARN System (see the Worksheets section) will ease the burden of reformatting the concepts into patient-friendly materials.

▓ INTERRELATIONSHIP WITH OTHER ELEMENTS OF THE LEARN SYSTEM

Building on the interactions between diet, activity, and restorative rest and sleep, The LEARN System leverages such interrelationships by optimizing each of the factors in a coordinated way. Improvements in one area such as dietary intake can be undone by little physical activity (the **A** component), and without restorative resting (the **R** component), there is little energy for activity or carrying on the pleasurable activities of daily life (the **L** component).

13

Giving Forward

Patients and their families are often grateful for the care and attention you have provided during their cancer treatment. With so many of the advances in cancer medicine made possible through philanthropy and sweat equity, patients and families are quite responsive to requests from *legitimate* organizations who fund or volunteer for clinical trials and patient-centered service delivery programs.

Under the current Health Insurance Portability and Accountability Act (HIPAA) regulation neither internal or extramural philanthropic requests *cannot be made* directly to your patient without your involvement unless a patient had explicitly consented cancer providers are the bridge to encourage fund-raising. This can bring up uncomfortable potential conflicts of interest particularly in regard to foundations or nonprofits to which we are connected. Technical as well as ethical questions arise.

Some practices advise patients at the time of initial consult or first visit that *selected* organizations may be contacting them unless they opt out of doing so, and a form or check box is provided on the registration form to do so. That is the simpler part.

The ethical dilemma is more challenging. Because we providers cannot guarantee patient outcomes, a gift to a cancer-related charity, foundation, or institution cannot be viewed as a way to ensure successful care, or that a response will be better than it will be. One smart patient, a meteorologist, compared the situation to the public making donations in the hopes of influencing weather patterns over a holiday weekend—a smart analogy. With many of our hospitals offering *concierge* services, including fancier rooms and higher quality food, such gifts are no longer a vehicle to a private room or a second desert on a patient's dinner tray. Through written material or discussion, *the intent of the donation is made explicit*, such as support clinical trails or patient services grants, such as transportation to and from treatment. Statements of appreciation and affirmations that such kindnesses will not affect a patient's care can be made if it is in your comfort zone. Corporate Compliance officers differ in their advice to providers about the necessity of such notice.

Patients who do not have the means to make monetary donations have a myriad of opportunities to donate time and effort through community organizations, houses of worship, your hospital's volunteer office, or cancer-related agencies. Their efforts to help with mailings, phone calls, at walks, races, or even doing friendly visits with the proper training are just a few ways patients can "give back" and "give forward" without financial obligation.

Families likewise show their appreciation after a patient has died from cancer by directing memorial donations. You, your practice, or your institution may have thought through a way to direct these requests. They can make us uncomfortable because the patient did not get better, and that's what we were supposed to do all along. The insightful weatherman further commented that because he cannot drive the weather, he can deliver an accurate forecast in the best way possible, and that he has learned to neither take credit nor blame when it's sunny or stormy. He has learned that people appreciate what he *can do*. Message well delivered to cancer providers!

Giving forward in whatever way is possible helps complete the circle for providers, patients, and families. Help continue these traditions.

Patient and Family Worksheets

WHAT IS IMPORTANT TO ME

I believe that life is precious and I want to continue living as well as I can for as long as I can.

At the time of my cancer diagnosis, I want to go through all of the necessary consultations and tests to determine, with the best medical expertise and judgment available:

- The kind of cancer I have: _____
- Where it is:
  - ❑ Locally advanced (where it started)
  - ❑ Lymph nodes
  - ❑ Other body systems; locations: _____
  _____

With treatment, it is my understanding that:

- ❑ I can be cancer-free for five years or more.
- ❑ I will likely need to be more treatment within the next five years.
- ❑ I will be on maintenance treatment for the rest of my life.

CHOOSE ONE (1) OF THE FOLLOWING:

❑ I am willing to do anything and everything necessary to control my cancer.

❑ I am interested in preserving my quality of life as well as surviving my cancer. With each proposed change in my treatment plan, please save a few minutes so we can discuss the benefit of the treatment and how I can expect to feel.

❑ I am more interested in preserving my quality of life if it is unlikely for me to survive my cancer for more than:

      ❑ 3 months   ❑ 6 months   ❑ 1 year   ❑ 2 years

❑ I am first and foremost interested in preserving my quality of life. If I do not get treatment or get abbreviated treatment, how will I feel?

_____

_____

CHOOSE ONE (1) OF THE FOLLOWING:

Whether my cancer responds to treatment or not, please be:

    ❑ as *optimistic* as possible in your advice

    ❑ as *pessimistic* as possible in your advice

    ❑ as *realistic* as possible in your advice

I think of myself as **strong** or **resilient**

    ❑ all of the time

    ❑ sometimes

    ❑ never

The worst thing in my life I have been through so far is:

_____

_____

_____

_____

_____

I got through it by doing the following:

_____

_____

_____

_____

_____

Here is other information you need to know about me and my family so that we can make the best possible decisions about my care:

_____

_____

_____

_____

_____

The answers to these questions are best supplemented by decisions regarding emergencies that may or may not happen in the course of cancer treatment. Each state has specific (and differing) laws regarding Health Care Power of Attorney, Living Will or Health Care Proxy forms and policies. One of the most useful forms to read, think about and complete is *Five Wishes*, produced by a private organization, *Aging With Dignity*. Find them at www.agingwithdignity.org or call 888-594-7743. *Five Wishes* adds to the depth of discussion.

FAMILY HISTORY FORM

Patient Name: _____ D.O.B._____ Today's Date: _____

Directions: Please list **all** of your <u>biological</u> (blood) relatives **below including those who have not had cancer. If someone is deceased, please put an asterisk** (*) in the age column next to the age at death. Use an additional page if you need extra space. You may not know each piece of information we are asking for. If you are unsure of something, give your best guess and put a question mark (?) next to it. It may be helpful to contact family members who may know additional information, but if this is not possible, we will do our best with the information you can give us.

<u>Relationship to You</u>	<u>Name or initials</u>	<u>Current age or age at death (mark* if deceased)</u>	<u>Date of birth (approximate if unsure)</u>	<u>Cancer type (s)</u> If person has not had cancer, leave blank.	<u>Age at cancer diagnosis</u>
<u>Your Children</u>	List your children below. In the first column, circle son or daughter for each child.				
Son / Daughter					
Son / Daughter					
Son / Daughter					
Son / Daughter					
Son / Daughter					
Son / Daughter					
<u>Your Brothers and Sisters</u>	List each of your brothers and sisters below. If half-sibling, specify which parent you share.				
Brother / Sister					
Brother / Sister					
Brother / Sister					
Brother / Sister					
Brother / Sister					
Brother / Sister					
<u>Nieces/Nephews</u>	List any of your nephews or nieces **IF** they have had cancer				
Niece / Nephew					
Niece / Nephew					
Niece / Nephew					
Niece / Nephew					

* Reprinted with permission: Norris Cotton Cancer Center, New Hampshire.

Patient Name: _____ D.O.B._____ Today's Date: _____

MOTHER'S SIDE OF THE FAMILY

Relationship to You	Name or initials	Current age or age at death (mark* if deceased)	Date of birth (approximate if unsure)	Cancer type (s) If person has not had cancer, leave blank.	Age at cancer diagnosis
Mother					
Mother's mother					
Mother's father					
Mother's Brothers/Sisters:	List each of you mother's brothers and sisters (your aunts and uncles) below, even if they did not have cancer. Circle aunt or uncle in the first column for each person.				
Aunt / Uncle					
Aunt / Uncle					
Aunt / Uncle					
Aunt / Uncle					
Aunt / Uncle					
Aunt / Uncle					
Aunt / Uncle					
Aunt / Uncle					
Aunt / Uncle					
Cousins	List any cousins on your mother's side <u>who have had cancer.</u> Specify who is his/her parent in the first column, i.e. Alice's daughter.				
Distant Relatives	List more distant relatives (i.e. great-aunts/uncles or great-grandparents) who had cancer. Specify how you are related in the first column, i.e. my mother's father's sister (great-aunt)				

* Reprinted with permission: Norris Cotton Cancer Center, New Hampshire.

Patient Name: _____ D.O.B. _____ Today's Date: _____

FATHER'S SIDE OF THE FAMILY

Relationship to You	Name or initials	Current age or age at death (mark* if deceased)	Date of birth (approximate if unsure)	Cancer type (s) If person has not had cancer, leave blank.	Age at cancer diagnosis
Father					
Father's mother					
Father's father					
Father's Brothers/Sisters	List each of you father's brothers and sisters (your aunts and uncles) below, even if they did not have cancer. Circle aunt or uncle in the first column for each person.				
Aunt / Uncle					
Aunt / Uncle					
Aunt / Uncle					
Aunt / Uncle					
Aunt / Uncle					
Aunt / Uncle					
Aunt / Uncle					
Aunt / Uncle					
Aunt / Uncle					
Cousins	List any cousins on your father's side who have had cancer. Specify who is his/her parent in the first column, i.e. Alice's daughter.				
Distant Relatives	List more distant relatives (i.e. great-aunts/uncles or great-grandparents) who had cancer. Specify how you are related in the first column, i.e. my father's mother's sister (great-aunt)				

* Reprinted with permission: Norris Cotton Cancer Center, New Hampshire.

IMPORTANT REVELATIONS TO MY TREATMENT TEAM

Please complete as many of the items that pertain to you and your family. Some of this information may be personal or embarrassing. Being candid will ease your treatment so that your needs can be best anticipated.

PART 1

Personal information:

I am the kind of person who likes *a lot/little* information.

Family history of important conditions that will affect my treatment:

Cancer (type, age) (For more detailed family history, see Family History Form)

Serious depression (even if never treated)

Significant drinking or drug (substance abuse problems)

Conditions important to consider during cancer treatment (see worksheet):

Motion sickness (trains, planes, car, bus)

Comfort level in closed spaces

Nausea/vomiting during pregnancy

Reactions to pain medicines if used in past

Reactions to steroid medicines if used in past

History of serious depression (even if never treated)

Authentic estimate of use of tobacco products

Authentic estimate of use of alcoholic beverages

IMPORTANT REVELATIONS TO MY TREATMENT TEAM

Use this checklist to prepare for your Initial Consultation. Its purpose is to have you think in advance about the information you may be asked.

PART 2

List of all the medicines I take: prescriptions; over-the-counter medications; vitamin, mineral, or nutritional supplements

_____

_____

Past illnesses and treatments

_____

_____

List all surgeries: type, date. Reactions to coming out of anesthesia (no one does it well).

_____

_____

Allergies (serious reactions with hives, rash, wheezing, or couldn't breathe)

_____

_____

Side effects I commonly get from medications (not the same as allergies)

_____

_____

❑ I am the kind of person who needs (a lot/little) information to make decisions.

❑ I want to be included in the decision-making process or I want to be given the resulting decision. If not myself, I trust _____ to speak for me.

❑ In my family, I suspect or am sure that these people had cancer and what kind. (See "Family History Form")

❑ I become frightened in closed spaces.

❑ I get train, car, bus, or plane sick regularly.

❑ When I was pregnant, I had bad nausea and/or vomiting during the early part of the pregnancy.

❑ I have regularly used strong "narcotic" opioid pain medicine for periods of time at significant doses when younger. I got "high" when I used them for pain relief. (yes/no; yes/no).

❑ I regularly used marijuana as a teenager or young adult. It did/did not make me "high."

❑ *Social drinking* to me means:_____.

❑ I do/do not get drunk regularly where I pass out or get mean.

❑ A close blood relative of mine (not someone who married into the family) has serious drinking or drug problems.

❑ I remember when my mother went through menopause and it was easy/hard.

❑ I have had periods of depression where I took to bed and couldn't function, whether they were treated or not.

❑ I have close blood relatives who had similar experiences.

❑ In my lifetime, the worst thing I have been through was: _____ and this is what I did to get through:_____

QUESTIONS I WANT ANSWERED

How will I feel?

Will I recover and be myself?

What will the treatment include?

Can I continue to work?

How can I arrange for a second opinion? (No offense, please, but this is serious and I need to know.)

Who can help with my kids? Will I need help at home?

What do I need to do during my treatment? Eating, exercise?

What will be affected by the cancer and by the treatments?

What about vitamins and supplements?

What are *clinical trials*?

What is important to me now?

What do I have to do to get better?

When will I feel OK again? Will I be the same?

Will the cancer come back?

Is it familial?

What do my family and friends need to know?

Will I be able to forget all of what is happening?

How long will I need follow-up care? What will it be?

Will I be OK?

What if nothing works?

What will happen if I get sicker?

Will you stick by me if treatment does not work?

How...and when will I die?

MY WEEKLY RECOVERY PLANNER
Using The LEARN System®

☐ post-operative   ☐ right after treatment

    ☐ chemotherapy ☐ radiation therapy   ☐ more than three months after treatment

    ☐ combinations of above

Living	Do:
	Done:
Education	Do:
	Done:
Activity	Do:
	Done:
Rest	Do:
	Done:
Nutrition	Do:
	Done:

DISTRESS THERMOMETER

Name:_____

Date: _____

Before you see your Nurse/Doctor, please complete this form. We would like to know how you are feeling and your concerns.

FIRST:
Please circle the number (0-10) that best describes *how much distress* you have been experiencing in the past week including today.

[name label]

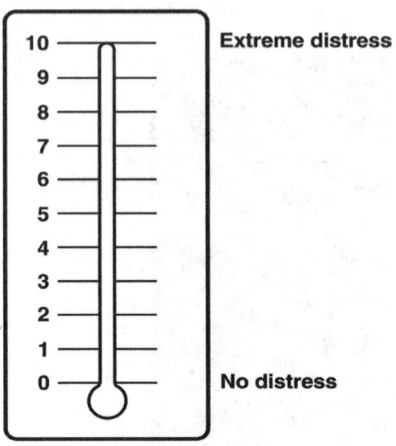

10 — Extreme distress
9
8
7
6
5
4
3
2
1
0 — No distress

THEN: Please indicate WHICH of the following is a cause of distress. A staff member may call you to follow-up. At what telephone number would you like to be called?_____

Practical
- ☐ Housing
- ☐ Insurance
- ☐ Work/school
- ☐ Transportation
- ☐ Child care

Family
- ☐ Dealing with partner
- ☐ Dealing with children

Emotional
- ☐ Worry
- ☐ Fears
- ☐ Sadness
- ☐ Depression
- ☐ Nervousness

Spiritual/Religious
- ☐ Relating to God
- ☐ Loss of faith

Physical
- ☐ Pain
- ☐ Nausea
- ☐ Fatigue [RN/MD: Hg:___ Hct:___]
- ☐ Sleep
- ☐ Getting around
- ☐ Bathing/dressing
- ☐ Breathing
- ☐ Mouth sores
- ☐ Eating
- ☐ Indigestion
- ☐ Constipation
- ☐ Diarrhea
- ☐ Changes in urination
- ☐ Fevers
- ☐ Skin dry/itchy
- ☐ Nose dry/congested
- ☐ Tingling in hands/feet
- ☐ Feeling swollen
- ☐ Sexual
- ☐ Legal

Other: _____

MY RECOVERY PLAN COMMUNICATOR
BREAST CANCER

Name: _____

Date: _____

Today and in the last three (3) days:

Energy: ❑ Good   ❑ Fair   ❑ Poor
Weight _____   ❑ Gain   ❑ Loss   Appetite: ❑ Good ❑ Fair ❑ Poor
Hot Flashes   ❑ Yes: _____ per day   ❑ No

Chemo: Date last given: _____
White cell count _____ Hemoglobin _____ Platelet count _____
[ ] erythropoeitin   [ ] filgastrim
❑ Nausea or vomiting
❑ Pins and needles or numbness anywhere, place: _____

Radiation: Skin reaction   ❑ yes   ❑ no   [ ] Aquaphor® [ ] Aloe Vera

[ ] Biafene® [ ] Silvadene® [ ] Other: _____

Surgery: Postoperative healing   ❑ good   ❑ not healing

Medications: name and dose: _____

_____

_____

Complementary therapies: _____

Pain 0–10 (0 = no pain; 10 = worst pain): _____
Swelling of breast: ❑ yes
Lymphedema: ❑ yes
Cough: ❑ yes

MY RECOVERY PLAN COMMUNICATOR
PROSTATE CANCER

Name: _____

Date: _____

Today and in the last three (3) days:

Energy: ❑ Good ❑ Fair ❑ Poor

Weight _____ ❑ Gain ❑ Loss   Appetite: ❑ Good ❑ Fair ❑ Poor

Urination: ❑ OK ❑ Frequently ❑ Need to go "right away"
❑ Can't urinate ❑ Blood in urine ❑ Pain

Hot Flashes ❑ Yes: ____ per day ❑ No

Chemo: White cell count _____ Hemoglobin _____ Platelet count _____
❑ Nausea or vomiting
❑ Pins and needles or numbness anywhere, place: _____

Radiation: Skin reaction ❑ yes ❑ no   Diarrhea ❑ yes ❑ no

Surgery: Postoperative healing ❑ good ❑ not healing

Medications: name and dose: _____

_____

_____

Complementary therapies: _____

Pain 0–10 (0 = no pain; 10 = worst pain):_____

Swelling of scrotum: ❑ yes

Lymphedema: ❑ yes

Cough: ❑ yes

MY RECOVERY PLAN COMMUNICATOR
LUNG OR ESOPHAGEAL CANCER

Name: _____

Date: _____

Today and in the last three (3) days:

Energy: ❑ Good ❑ Fair ❑ Poor

Weight _____ ❑ Gain ❑ Loss   Appetite: ❑ Good ❑ Fair ❑ Poor

Breathing: ❑ OK   Short of breath: ❑ all of the time ❑ walking around

❑ Cough: ❑ No ❑ Yes: ❑ with mucus/phlegm ❑ with blood

❑ white "cheesy" spots in mucus ❑ dry

❑ Pain ❑ on breathing ❑ other part of body: name where: _____

❑ Difficulty swallowing

Skin reaction ❑ yes ❑ no [ ] Aquaphor® [ ] Aloe Vera [ ] Biafene®
[ ] Silvadene® [ ] Other: _____

❑ Pins and needles or numbness anywhere, place(s): _____

❑ Palpitations

Chemo: White cell count _____ Hemoglobin _____ Platelet count _____

❑ Nausea or vomiting

Radiation: Skin reaction ❑ yes ❑ no   Diarrhea ❑ yes ❑ no

Surgery: Postoperative healing ❑ good ❑ not healing

Medications: name and dose: _____

_____

_____

Complementary therapies: _____

Pain 0–10 (0 = no pain; 10 = worst pain): _____

Swelling of neck: ❑ yes

Lymphedema: ❑ yes

Cough: ❑ yes

MY RECOVERY PLAN COMMUNICATOR
COLON, RECTAL, STOMACH, OR PANCREATIC CANCER

Name: _____

Date: _____

Today and in the last three (3) days:

Energy: ❑ Good ❑ Fair ❑ Poor

Weight _____ ❑ Gain ❑ Loss Appetite: ❑ Good ❑ Fair ❑ Poor

Breathing: ❑ OK Short of breath: ❑ all of the time ❑ walking around

Bowel movements: ❑ Well formed ❑ Loose (diarrhea) ❑ Soft
❑ Hard (constipated)

Skin reaction ❑ yes ❑ no [ ] Aquaphor® [ ] Aloe Vera [ ] Biafene®
[ ] Silvadene® [ ] Other: _____

❑ Pain ❑ No ❑ Yes: where: _____ when: ❑ sitting ❑ lying down on back

❑ Pins and needles, coldness or numbness anywhere, place: _____

Chemo: White cell count _____Hemoglobin _____ Platelet count _____
❑ Nausea or vomiting

Radiation: Skin reaction ❑ yes ❑ no

Surgery: Postoperative healing ❑ good ❑ not healing

Medications: name and dose: _____

_____

_____

Complementary therapies: _____

Pain 0–10 (0 = no pain; 10 = worst pain): _____

Swelling of abdomen or legs: ❑ yes

Lymphedema: ❑ yes

Cough: ❑ yes

MY RECOVERY PLAN COMMUNICATOR
OVARIAN, CERVICAL, OR UTERINE CANCER

Name: _____

Date: _____

Today and in the last three (3) days:

Energy: ❑ Good ❑ Fair ❑ Poor

Weight _____ ❑ Gain ❑ Loss   Appetite: ❑ Good ❑ Fair ❑ Poor

Vaginal bleeding: ❑ No ❑ Yes: number of pads used in 24 hours: ____

Skin reaction ❑ yes ❑ no [ ] Aquaphor® [ ] Aloe Vera [ ] Biafene® [ ] Silvadene® [ ] Other: _____

Breathing: ❑ OK Short of breath: ❑ all of the time ❑ walking around

Bowel movements: ❑ Well formed ❑ Loose (diarrhea) ❑ Soft ❑ Hard (constipated)

Urination: ❑ OK ❑ Frequently ❑ Need to go "right away" ❑ Can't urinate ❑ Blood in urine ❑ Pain

Hot Flashes ❑ Yes: ____ per day ❑ No

❑ Pain ❑ No ❑ Yes: where: _____ when: ❑ sitting ❑ lying down on back

❑ Pins and needles, coldness or numbness anywhere, place: _____

Chemo: White cell count _____ Hemoglobin _____ Platelet count _____
❑ Nausea or vomiting

Radiation: Skin reaction ❑ yes ❑ no

Surgery: Postoperative healing ❑ good ❑ not healing

Medications: name and dose: _____

_____

_____

Complementary therapies:_____

Pain 0–10 (0 = no pain; 10 = worst pain):_____

Swelling of abdomen or legs: ❑ yes

Lymphedema: ❑ yes

Cough: ❑ yes

MY RECOVERY PLAN COMMUNICATOR
HEAD AND NECK CANCER

Name: _____

Date: _____

Today and in the last three (3) days:

Energy: ❑ Good ❑ Fair ❑ Poor
Weight _____ ❑ Gain ❑ Loss Appetite: ❑ Good ❑ Fair ❑ Poor
Skin reaction ❑ yes ❑ no [ ] Aquaphor® [ ] Aloe Vera [ ] Biafene®
[ ] Silvadene® [ ] Other: _____
Breathing: ❑ OK Short of breath: ❑ all of the time ❑ walking around
Swallowing: ❑ OK ❑ Painful ❑ Can't
Talking: ❑ OK ❑ Painful ❑ Can't
Mouth: ❑ Too dry ❑ Too much mucous ❑ Inflamed ❑ Can't chew
❑ Lockjaw
Taste: ❑ None ❑ Things don't taste like they are supposed to taste
Voice: ❑ Voice changes ❑ Hoarse
❑ Cough: ❑ No ❑ Yes: ❑ with mucus/phlegm ❑ with blood
❑ white "cheesy" spots in mucus ❑ dry
Bowel movements: ❑ Well formed ❑ Loose (diarrhea) ❑ Soft
❑ Hard (constipated)
❑ Pain ❑ No ❑ Yes: where: _____ when: ❑ sitting ❑ lying down on back
❑ Pins and needles, coldness or numbness anywhere, place: _____

Chemo: White cell count _____ Hemoglobin _____ Platelet count _____
❑ Nausea or vomiting

Radiation: Skin reaction ❑ yes ❑ no

Surgery: Postoperative healing ❑ good ❑ not healing

Medications: name and dose: _____

_____

_____

Complementary therapies: _____

Pain 0–10 (0 = no pain; 10 = worst pain): _____
Swelling of face or neck: ❑ yes
Lymphedema: ❑ yes
Cough: ❑ yes

148

MY RECOVERY PLAN COMMUNICATOR
KIDNEY OR BLADDER CANCER

Name: _____

Date: _____

Today and in the last three (3) days:

Energy:　　❏ Good　❏ Fair　❏ Poor

Weight _____　❏ Gain　❏ Loss　　Appetite:　❏ Good　❏ Fair　❏ Poor

Urination:　❏ OK　❏ Frequently　❏ Need to go "right away"
❏ Blood in urine　❏ Pain

Bowel movements:　❏ Well formed　❏ Loose (diarrhea)　❏ Soft
❏ Hard (constipated)

Breathing:　❏ OK　Short of breath:　❏ all of the time　❏ walking around

Swelling:　❏ legs　❏ hands

Skin reaction　❏ yes　❏ no [ ] Aquaphor® [ ] Aloe Vera [ ] Biafene®
[ ] Silvadene® [ ] Other: _____

Chemo: White cell count _____Hemoglobin _____ Platelet count _____
❏ Nausea or vomiting
❏ Pins and needles or numbness anywhere, place: _____

Radiation: Skin reaction　❏ yes　❏ no　Diarrhea　❏ yes　❏ no

Surgery: Postoperative healing　❏ good　❏ not healing

Medications: name and dose: _____

_____

_____

Complementary therapies: _____

Pain 0–10 (0 =no pain; 10 = worst pain): _____
Swelling of abdomen or legs:　❏ yes
Lymphedema:　❏ yes
Cough:　❏ yes

MY RECOVERY PLAN COMMUNICATOR
BRAIN OR SPINAL CORD CANCER

Name: _____

Date: _____

Today and in the last three (3) days:

Energy: ❑ Good ❑ Fair ❑ Poor
Weight _____ ❑ Gain ❑ Loss   Appetite: ❑ Good ❑ Fair ❑ Poor
Urination: ❑ OK ❑ Frequently ❑ Need to go "right away"
❑ Blood in urine ❑ Pain
Bowel movements: ❑ Well formed ❑ Loose (diarrhea) ❑ Soft
❑ Hard (constipated)

❑ Changes in ability to move: part of body: _____
❑ Involuntary movements ❑ seizure activity
❑ Changes in sensations: part of body: _____
❑ Changes in speech
❑ Change in ability to retain information

Chemo: White cell count _____Hemoglobin _____ Platelet count _____
❑ Nausea or vomiting
❑ Pins and needles or numbness anywhere, place: _____

Radiation: Skin reaction ❑ yes ❑ no   Diarrhea ❑ yes ❑ no

Surgery: Postoperative healing ❑ good ❑ not healing

Medications: name and dose: _____

_____

_____

Complementary therapies:_____

Pain 0–10 (0 = no pain; 10 = worst pain):_____
Swelling of head or neck: ❑ yes
Lymphedema: ❑ yes

150

Journal Page: Charting My Course

ENTERAL NUTRITION (TUBE FEEDING)

WHAT IS ENTERAL NUTRITION?

Enteral nutrition is using a feeding tube to help you get enough nutrition when you cannot eat well or are unable to eat. The feeding tube is placed very carefully into your stomach. It is called a *PEG* (percutaneous endoscopic gastrostomy). Sometimes, the doctors will place the tube in the area just past your stomach, called the jejunum. This is called a *PEJ* (percutaneous endoscopic jejunostomy). The doctor or nurse will show you how they put the tube in.

HOW DO I GET FOOD THROUGH A TUBE?

Once the tube is in the right place, liquid food is put down the tube. The food is like a shake and contains vitamins, minerals, and other nutrients your body needs. The food usually comes in cans, and the nutritionist will discuss how many to use per day to maintain good nutrition.

THESE ARE DIFFERENT WAYS TO USE THE PEG

Bolus Administration

The easiest way to give a feeding is called a bolus, which is all at once and is like eating a meal. Each can of feeding may take up to 15–30 minutes to go down the tube using a *syringe* or *gravity bag*. This kind of feeding is given four to six times a day, depending on how many cans you need. Specific instructions are given on the following pages.

Continuous Drip

This is when the feeding goes into the PEG tube for the entire day and/or night at a slow rate. A small, easy-to-use pump makes sure the right amount of food goes through the tube.

WHAT DO I NEED TO DO?

It's very important to keep the tube in the right place, so try to avoid pulling it or moving it by accident. You will need to give yourself regular feedings and water to *maintain your weight* and *get enough nutrition for energy and healing.*

Your nurse will show you how to take care of your tube and what to watch out for. Your supplies will be delivered to your home a few days after the PEG is placed.

Please make sure you ask any questions you have!

YOU AND YOUR FEEDING TUBE:
A READY REFERENCE GUIDE

TUBE TYPE: _____

APPEARANCE AND SITE CARE (DAILY)

Cleanse where tube exits skin and under the bumper with warm soap and water. Pat dry.

The site will usually have a dressing for the first 48 hours. Thin gauze pads may be used under the bumper after this.

Tube may become cloudy in appearance or develop black discoloration, which does *not* indicate a need for change of tube.

Scar tissue can develop around the tube, which is red and may bleed slightly if moved.

Secure the tube into the waistline of your pants or with a Spandage® to minimize its movement.

TUBE FEEDINGS

Formula: _____

Method: ❑ Syringe (Bolus) ❑ Gravity Bag (Bolus) ❑ Bag with Pump
(Continuous)

Amount & Frequency: _____

Medications

Some medications *cannot be crushed*—ask your health care team about your medication if you are unable to swallow pills. If you need to put your medication through the tube, be sure the pills are finely crushed and dissolved with warm water before you start. Always let a syringe full of water flow through the tube before and after the medication is given. *Do not push fluid through... let it flow in.*

THINGS TO WATCH FOR

Call the health care team right away if you have...

• A blocked tube or if tube slips out
• Worsening/increasing pain at PEG tube site for more than one week after placement
• Signs/symptoms of infection—excessive redness, swelling, unusual drainage, or foul smell
• Fever of 100.5 degrees or higher
• Leakage or excessive bleeding around tube (spots of blood on gauze pad is *not* a concern)
• Vomiting, diarrhea, dehydration, constipation, excess fullness, or tasting feeds in your mouth

PHONE NUMBERS

Please call if you have concerns or questions.

PHYSICIAN: _____

Phone #: _____

PHYSICIAN: _____

Phone #: _____

NURSE: _____

Phone #: _____

DIETITIAN: _____

Phone #: _____

SOCIAL WORKER: _____

Phone #: _____

VENDOR: _____

Phone #: _____

HOW TO GIVE YOURSELF A TUBE FEEDING: BEFORE STARTING THE FEEDING

Gather supplies: Formula can(s), feeding bag and/or syringe, and 1 cup (8 oz.) of water.

Wash hands with soap and water before setting up the feeding.

Rinse top of the can and shake well before opening. Cans should be *room temperature*.

Sit up in a chair or raise the head of bed (do not feed while lying down).

Attach syringe to your feeding tube and let 1/2 cup (4 oz.) lukewarm water flow in.

FEEDING PROCEDURE

If using a syringe:

Open the can.

Remove the plunger from the syringe, pinch the PEG closed with thumb and finger to avoid leaks and attach the syringe to the feeding tube securely.

Hold the syringe in one hand and pour the can contents into the syringe with the other, slowly filling the syringe but not to the very top. Let the liquid flow in on its own—*do not* use the plunger to push it through.

NOTE: To control the flow of feeding:

—Lowering the syringe will slow the rate of feeding.

—Raising the syringe will speed up the rate of feeding.

It takes about 15–30 minutes for one can to flow in by gravity, depending on the rate of feeding. If any discomfort occurs, discuss with your health care team.

After the feeding, use the syringe to flush your PEG tube again with 1/2 cup warm water, or more if instructed to do so.

Pinch the PEG closed, detach the syringe, and close the port on the PEG tube.

Avoid lying down for an hour after feeding to prevent heartburn or backflow.

Rinse and dry the syringe after each feeding.

If using a gravity bag:

The bag should be hung on the IV pole at least 18 inches above the level of your stomach.

Close the clamp on the feeding bag.

Open the can and pour contents into the bag.

Open the clamp on the feeding tube bag to let the liquid fill the tubing completely, then close the clamp (do this over the sink or garbage pail).

Pinch the PEG closed, open the port and attach the bag tubing securely to it.

Open the clamp to start the feeding.

NOTE: To control the flow of the feeding, roll the clamp up to go faster and down to go slower.

It takes about 20–30 minutes for one can of feeding to be absorbed, depending on the rate of feeding. If any discomfort occurs, discuss with your health care team.

After the feeding is complete, close the clamp on the feeding bag and pinch the PEG tube before removing the bag to prevent a leak.

Use the syringe to flush your PEG tube again with 1/2 cup (4oz.) warm water (or more as instructed).

Detach the syringe and close the port on the PEG tube.

Avoid lying down for an hour after feeding to prevent heartburn or backflow.

After each feeding, rinse the feeding bag and tubing with warm water until the water runs clear. Dry with a paper towel and store in a clean place until the next feeding.

WHAT I AM SUPPOSED TO BE EATING OR DRINKING WHEN I CAN'T EAT ANYTHING

Right after chemotherapy or during radiation therapy (involving the mouth, neck, and esophagus or if mouth sores develop from any treatment):

I FEEL TOO SICK OR NAUSEOUS. WHAT IF READING THIS MAKES ME NOT FEEL WELL?

Pass the worksheet to someone else to read who can help.

Ask your oncologist or oncology nurse if your regimen is highly emetogenic, moderately emetogenic or minimally emetogenic. The higher the chance of nausea and/or vomiting (emetogenesis), the longer it will take to move through the phases (1, 2, etc.). Some combinations will not cause much nausea the first few days due to the anti-nausea medication cocktail that accompanies it, others can show a surge 5–10 days afterward. Understand the usual pattern connected with your chemotherapy drugs and anti-nausea drugs so you can move through the Phases as quickly as possible.

Phase 1

You really need to make sure that fluids are moving in (and out). At a bare minimum. If it's early in the day (equivalent to breakfast time), try some juice of your choice, diluted with water. Half juice and half water. This will keep you from getting dehydrated (in any climate). A sports drink (Gatorade® and others) is fine. Put it in a sports cup with a straw, and sip a little bit at a time, so that the cup is emptied within a few hours or sooner. Optional addition to juice/water: 1/2 teaspoon of Morton's Lite Salt® or similar (or any potassium-based salt substitute) will replace some of the potassium your body loses, unless your oncologist or nurse tells you it is not necessary for you, based on the blood tests taken before chemotherapy (700 mg of potassium in 1/2 teaspoon is about 18 mEq of potassium).

Important Note: If your chemotherapy contained cis-platin or cyclophosphamide, this fluid is more than essential. Without it, the chemotherapy stays too long in your kidneys and bladder and is damaging.

For later in the day, clear broth of your choice (chicken, beef, vegetable) is ideal if that's the most complex food you can tolerate. If you have not added the Lite Salt to juice earlier in the day, add it to one of the cups of broth. Make it moderately warm. Or even cold if you are in a very hot climate. Sip a little at a time.

If you can tolerate, add some type of fiber, such as brown rice, whole wheat pasta (cooked way too much for general use so it is soft).

Thick or thin? *Although our first impulse is to reach for some water (how much more basic can we get?) as the first thing to swallow, it may be among the hardest choices due to the thin consistency. For any and all foods, thin foods can be made thicker with a commercially made product (Thick-it® or similar). Made of malto-dextrin and corn starch, such additives can be thought of as a "bridge" to regular consistency foods rather than an additive to use for a long time. Depending upon the food, unflavored gelatin may be a more healthful alternative. Gelatin is usually added right before eating as a thickener to hot foods or else the proteins are denatured by the heat and the food returns to its original consistency. It has a small amount of protein and no carbohydrate. To use gelatin effectively, sprinkle it into warm (not boiling water) so that it rests on the surface for 10–15 minutes, then mix the gelatin with the food to be thickened just before it is served or in the very last minutes of cooking.*

Continued

I FEEL A BIT HUNGRY. WHAT'S NEXT?

Phase 2

You've been able to tolerate the diluted juice and soup. Let's ramp up one small notch. Try a smoothie shake (see recipe or a commercially sold drink, such as Ensure Plus®, Boost®, or Nutren 1.5® and others. Compare labels to maximize proteins and minimize sugars to taste. Those with diabetes have other options, such as Glucerna® and others). Use the sports bottle, sip a bit at a time. Can be diluted, but more to drink. Use them as you can but continuously.

Smoothie Shake *(courtesy of Bridget Bennett, MS, RD)*

Basic Ingredients:

- 1 cup any liquid (whole milk, soy milk, rice milk, almond milk, etc.; use more than 1 cup if needed to blend.)
- 2 tablespoons protein powder (any type: soy, whey, egg)
- 1 tablespoon canola, olive or other oil
- 1 banana or other fresh or frozen fruit

For added protein, calories, and fiber, the following items can also be added:

- 1/2 cup plain or flavored organic yogurt, soy yogurt or soft tofu
- 1 tablespoon peanut butter, almond butter, cashew butter
- 1 tablespoon ground flaxseeds (optional)

Instructions:

- Blend all of the ingredients together to your desired consistency.
- Add additional liquid or ice to the blender if needed to thin out consistency for better blending. You may need more or less liquid to make the mixture blend.
- Add flavors or extracts if desired.
- Be creative.
- Store any excess in the refrigerator & give a quick re-blend before drinking.

Variation: See *Bridget's Basic Recipe* to create on your own.

MAN (WOMAN) DOES NOT LIVE BY SMOOTHIES ALONE. I NEED MORE!

Phase 3

Move up to something a little more substantial. Smooth warm cereals work well and provide protein, complex carbohydrates and fiber.

Early in the day: *Oatmeal, Cream of Wheat,* or *Cream of Rice* flavored with a small amount of butter, honey, and/or fresh fruit.

If you are getting radiation to the mouth, neck or chest, choose the smoothest type (oatmeal that is constantly stirred when made so it is creamier).

Later in the day: *Polenta* can be made the same way or with more savory flavoring as lunch or dinner. Can use olive oil instead of butter.

Options besides cornmeal (polenta): *buckwheat groats, couscous, pastina* (very small pasta pieces). *Quinoa* is actually not a grain but the seed of a leafy plant related to spinach. It has more protein than other carbohydrate grains, and cooks up into a smooth cereal-like consistency that adopts the flavors of the foods that are combined with it.

PRINCIPLES OF FLAVORING AFTER CHEMOTHERAPY OR DURING RADIATION THERAPY (OF THE MOUTH, NECK, OR CHEST)

Think of the taste buds having four primary flavors that work together to form the thousands of flavors we experience (similar to colors where all colors are mixtures of the primary colors: red, blue and yellow): bitter, acid, sweet, salty, and umami. All of the taste buds will not go into suspended animation at once, so familiar foods may taste odd (bitter dessert instead of sweet, vinegar sweet instead of bitter, etc.).

To compensate, make the flavor that is missing more intense to see if it breaks through the taste buds that are still functioning, even if not at capacity OR concentrate on foods that expectedly taste like the flavors you *can* taste.

For later in the day eating, can add the same broths used previously (may think about fish stock, based upon food preferences in addition to vegetable, chicken or beef). Some people like to graduate to tomato bases, even starting with tomato juices (or a vegetable fortified one, like V-8® and others). Adding some mild cheese can also vary the taste with additional protein. Plain cheeses (low-fat cottage cheese or ricotta cheese) are the easiest to tolerate, then can graduate to aged, sharper cheeses (cheddar, parmesan or Romano types). Using a stock made from mushrooms (Portobello, for example) adds even a different flavor dimension.

Can even move into whole wheat pasta (whole wheat better than regular, but regular will do) that is cooked on the softer side—unless you're up to al dente—and made slippery with mild sauces, or even butter-flavored olive oils with herbs, tomato sauces, or cheese sauces (from bland to spicy based upon food preferences and tasting abilities).

I'M TOO TIRED TO CHEW AND EAT REGULAR FOOD. IDEAS?

Phase 4

Use the vegetable, chicken, beef or fish stocks to make thicker soups. Think about what are really favorites—this is not hospital food. Even favorites become boring day after day, and if the goal is proper nutrition, then boring is counterproductive. Vary the recipes between the basic stocks and add whatever you like. Well-cooked lean meats, chicken, turkey or soft poached fish matched with the stock flavor of your choice. Add vegetables of as many different colors as you can. Cook well. At first, be prepared to put the resulting soup in a blender or food processor if it seems like too much work to chew and swallow, or the consistency is irritating to the mouth or esophagus. Judge what size pieces are tolerable, and may reach the point where well-cooked soft contents are fine on their own without processing.

Soft foods that are *slicked* with an oil or liquid. Think about poached egg whites (OK; whole eggs of course; unless your cholesterol levels were dangerously high before the cancer) with butter or butter-flavored oils. Some naturally slippery foods may be quite a treat (even something like a steamed oyster or clam; raw is not a good idea due to the risk of infection) slathered in a sauce or butter/oil.

For a treat, add puddings in the flavors you like, ice cream (or sorbets, unless high blood sugars or hypoglycemic reactions make such a load of simple sugars a bad idea). To be the most careful, many brands of commercially prepared ice cream come in *no sugar added* formulations. (Can use them on their own or add to smoothie drinks.)

Vary phases 1, 2, 3, and 4 during treatment, based upon tolerance. Of course, be prepared to jump back to phase 1 foods with each chemotherapy cycle, then advance as tolerated.

MORE THAN CHIPS AND CANDY...GOOD SNACKS?

Snacks (courtesy of Bridget Bennett, MS, RD):

Each of these has about 1 serving of carb and 1–2 oz. protein, for a nice balance.

¼ cups nuts and dried fruit or a piece of fresh fruit, take with lots of water or herbal tea

1 tablespoon natural peanut butter spread on 2–3 Ryvita crackers (high fiber)

1 low-fat string cheese with any piece of fresh fruit

1/3 cup low-fat cottage cheese with 1 cup fruit salad

1 low-fat yogurt, add some nuts to it

1 Balance bar or Luna Bar (has protein, vitamins/minerals, and carbs) if you're craving sweet

Small cup of bean or chicken soup if you're craving savory

Tips for Adding Calories

■ Eat snacks between meals and at bedtime—choose peanut butter, hummus or bean dip, dried fruit and nuts if tolerated, custards, string cheese, drinkable yogurt, smoothies, and so forth.

■ Add olive oil or butter to warm prepared dishes such as eggs, sweet potatoes, soups, pasta, and so forth.

■ Drink high-calorie beverages such as smoothies, shakes, nectars, juice, whole milk, and nutritional supplements, which have more calories than water, coffee, or tea.

■ Add avocado or mayonnaise to dishes and use other sauces liberally to moisten foods.

■ Make your own shakes with whole or soy milk, fruit, peanut butter, frozen yogurt, ice cream, protein powder, honey, and so forth.

■ Substitute milk for water when making soups, pudding, and warm cereals such as oatmeal or grits.

Tips for Adding Protein

■ High protein foods include meat, poultry, fish, eggs, beans, cheese, tofu, and other soy products as well as most dairy products. Whole grains, such as quinoa, bulgur, and barley, also contain protein. Nuts, nut butters, and seeds contain protein as well as healthy fats.

■ Add protein powder (whey, egg, or soy based) or dry milk powder to foods and drinks such as soups, smoothies, milkshakes, casseroles, sauces, cooked cereals, eggs, and mashed potatoes.

■ Blend chopped hard-cooked eggs into soups or casseroles. DON'T EAT RAW EGGS.

■ Mash cooked beans and use as a dip or spread.

■ Add canned or cooked beans to salads or rice or use as a side dish.

■ Add grated cheese to top warm dishes such as eggs, soups, casseroles, and vegetables.

■ Add tofu to soups or salads or blend into liquids (soft tofu).

■ Use 4 percent cottage cheese as a side dish or with fruit.

■ Sprinkle flaxseed meal or wheat germ to vegetables, cereal, ice cream, or yogurt. A word of caution: Uncooked vegetables and unwashed fruits can harbor bacteria. Best to peel or wash fruits and vegetables well, including those labeled, "pre-washed".

Bridget Bennett, MS, RD, is an Oncology Nutritionist working with patients with cancer and their families for many years. She serves as the senior Oncology Nutritionist at the Continuum Cancer Centers of New York.

Bridget is reluctant to admit that her movie career skyrocketed with her appearance as the dietician in Super Size Me, *a film about the fast-food industry.*

Bridget's Basic Recipe

Use the following recipe for the base, meaning a *very plain* liquid, to which you may add foods.

Basic Recipe	Calories	Protein	Carbohydrate	Fat
Whole milk 1 cup	150	8 g	12 g	8 g
Canola oil, olive oil, etc. 1 tablespoon	120	0	0	14 (unsat.)
Protein powder **(whey, soy, egg)** 1 scoop: varied, see label	100	20 g	1 g	1 g
Total =	370	28 g	13 g	23 g

To this base an endless variety of additions can be added and blended in as desired, based on a person's taste, tolerance, and nutritional needs.

Nutritional Breakdown

The basic recipe will have about 300–400 calories and 20–30 grams of protein per 1 cup or so, but these values will increase with any additions you make to your own personal smoothie!

"THE IDEAL COUPLE"

An ideal pairing of rustic whole wheat bread and omega-3 fatty acid fish oils* together can supply good complex carbohydrates and the omega-3s. It's like eating in a fine restaurant where the butter brought with the bread has been switched to flavored olive oil. The added calories plus fiber and oil lubrication against constipation makes this snack an *ideal couple.*

Make sure the *rustic* whole what bread actually contains whole wheat flour, not just various seeds added to make it appear healthy.

Add a small amount of the herb of your choice (rosemary is a favorite), and you'll almost think you're in Tuscany (maybe).

* There are a variety of omega-3 oils on the market, some are already flavored (lemon flavored oil goes great with the rosemary). On the Internet, use your favorite search engine for "omega 3 oils" or "omega 3 oils lemon" to see what is available and where you can purchase it. You can certainly mix omega-3 oils with some olive oil for taste, but keep the majority as omega-3.

I'VE RECOVERED ENOUGH TO GET BACK TO REGULAR FOODS. I MADE THE PROMISE TO EAT MORE HEALTHFULLY. WHERE CAN I GET INSPIRATION? (IS PHASE 5 THE LAST PHASE?)

Dana's Recipes

Dana Jacobi, a well-respected chef, has been working with the special needs of the cancer community for many years. She writes a column for the American Institute for Cancer Research (AICR) and is the author of a number of creative, practical, and beautiful books: Cook & Freeze: 150 Delicious Dishes to Serve Now and Later, Dana's Market Basket, *and* The 12 Best Foods Cookbook: Over 200 Recipes Featuring the 12 Healthiest Foods.

Dana's columns are available through the AICR at www.aicr.org, along with sound nutritional information. Dana's additional work can be viewed at www.dana-jacobi.com and by blogging at www.danasmarketbasket.com.

The following suggestions may even be considered phase 5, since their flavors and textures are more complex. These recipes provide examples of good foods that can be prepared nutritiously at the end of treatment and further into survivorship to counteract our reliance on processed foods with enriched flour and sugar products. The corn pudding requires more time in the kitchen. Many more appear in Dana's books, and serve as examples of how we can alter our diet without sacrificing taste.

Cocoa Nutty Smoothie

Chocoholics love this rich smoothie. It offers a perfect balance of cocoa flavor, peanut butter, and sweetness from a frozen banana. Serves 1.

1 cup chocolate milk (almond, hemp, or coconut can be substituted for dairy milk)

1 small banana, sliced and frozen

2 tablespoons natural smooth peanut butter

2 tablespoons unsweetened cocoa powder

2 ice cubes

1. Combine the milk, banana, peanut butter, and cocoa in a blender. Blend until creamy. With the blender running, add the ice cubes and blend until smooth. Pour into a tall glass and serve.

California Date Shake

Southern Californians have long enjoyed this thick, creamy milk shake. The secret to making this fiber-rich smooth drink is using moist Medjool dates and blending them with hot water before adding the other ingredients. A touch of coffee adds an interesting note, if you wish. Serves 2.

1/2 cup chopped, pitted Medjool dates (4–6 dates)
1 cup vanilla ice cream or frozen yogurt
1 cup milk
1/2 teaspoon ground cinnamon
4 ice cubes

1. Place the dates and 1/2 cup boiling water in a blender, and whirl to purée.
2. Add the frozen yogurt, milk, cinnamon, and ice cubes. Whirl until the ice is blended. Divide between two tall glasses and drink immediately.

Baked Oatmeal

This is a great way to enjoy oatmeal. Dried fruits and an apple make this a more complete breakfast. Serves 4.

1-3/4 cups milk
1 tablespoon unsalted butter
1/8 teaspoon salt
1 cup old-fashioned rolled oats
1/4 cup dried apricots
1/4 cup raisins
3 tablespoon lightly packed brown sugar, divided
1/2 Golden Delicious apple, peeled
3 tablespoons chopped walnuts

1. Preheat the oven to 350°F.
2. In a 2-quart microwaveable, ovenproof casserole, heat the milk and butter until the milk steams. Mix in the salt and oats and set aside.
3. Chop the apricots. Mix the apricots, raisins, and 1 tablespoon of the sugar into the oats. Shred the apple into the oats and mix to combine.
4. Bake the oats, uncovered, for 15 minutes. Stir, then top with the remaining sugar and the nuts. Bake 15 minutes longer, or until the oats are chewy. Divide the oatmeal among four bowls. Serve immediately, accompanied by a pitcher of cold milk.

Baked Corn Pudding

This colorful casserole is equally good as a meatless main course or as a side dish with pork chops or roast chicken or pork chops. Serves 6–8.

1/2 cup stone-ground yellow corn meal

1/2 cup all-purpose flour

1 teaspoon baking powder

2 tablespoon sugar

1 small onion, chopped

1/2 cup chopped scallions, green and white parts

4 tablespoons unsalted butter, melted

1 can (15¼ oz.) corn, drained

1 can (14¾ oz.) creamed corn

1 large egg, beaten

1 cup shredded cheddar cheese, divided

1/2 teaspoon salt

1/8 teaspoon freshly ground pepper

1 (4 oz.) can green chiles, drained

1. Preheat the oven to 350°F. Coat an 8-inch square baking dish with cooking spray and set aside.
2. In a bowl, combine the corn meal, flour, baking powder, and sugar, and set aside.
3. Place onions and scallions in strainer and plunge them into a medium pot of boiling water for 30 seconds. Cool the vegetables under cold running water, drain very well, and set aside.
4. In large mixing bowl, combine the corn, creamed corn, egg, and butter. Add the dry ingredients and mix just to combine. Mix in the onions, scallions and 1/2 cup of the cheese. Spread the pudding in prepared baking dish. Sprinkle the remaining 1/2 cup cheese over top of pudding.
5. Bake the casserole for 40 minutes, until the pudding is puffed and golden on top and a knife inserted into the center comes out clean. Cool the pudding on a wire rack for 15 minutes before serving.

Continued

Three Bean Salad with Mustard Dressing

Using mayonnaise and yogurt to make a creamy dressing gives this popular salad a different twist. Serves 4.

1 cup canned chickpeas, rinsed and drained

1 cup canned Great Northern beans, rinsed and drained

1 cup canned kidney, rinsed and drained

1/2 cup finely chopped red onion

2 tablespoons yogurt

1 tablespoon mayonnaise

1 tablespoon Dijon-style mustard

1 teaspoon white vinegar

2 dashes hot pepper sauce

1/2 teaspoon salt

1/4 teaspoon ground black pepper

2 teaspoons extra virgin olive oil

1/2 cup chopped fresh dill or flat-leaf parsley

1. In a mixing bowl, combine the drained beans with the onion.
2. For the dressing, whisk together the yogurt, mayonnaise, mustard, vinegar, hot sauce, salt and pepper. Continuing to whisk, drizzle in the oil. Add the dressing to the beans and mix to combine. If serving immediately, mix in the dill or parsley. Or, cover the dressed beans and refrigerate for up to 8 hours, and add the herbs just before serving.

Share Your Ideas!

These recipes are here for your convenience and immediate use but should also serve as a springboard for creativity.

To *Give Forward* to future generations of patients and their caregivers, share your successes on   www.cancerknowanddo.com.

TRUSTED INTERNET SITES

For general cancer information:

American Cancer Society: www.cancer.org

American Society of Clinical Oncology: www.asco.org

National Cancer Institute :   www.cancer.gov

National Comprehensive Cancer Network (especially patient guides to professional guidelines):   www.nccn.org

For specialty groups:

American Cancer Society: www.cancer.org

American Psychosocial Oncology Society: www.apos-society.org

American Society of Clinical Oncology: www.asco.org

American Society for Radiation Oncology: www.astro.org

The Bladder Cancer Advocacy Network: www.bcan.org

Breast Cancer Network for Strength: www.networkofstrength.org

Cancer*Care*:   www.cancercare.org

The Children's Cause for Cancer Advocacy: www.childrenscause.org

Coalition of Cancer Cooperative Groups: www.cancertrialshelp.org

C-3: Colorectal Cancer Coalition: www.FightColorectalCancer.org

Education Network to Advance Cancer Clinical Trials: www.enacct.org

International Myeloma Foundation: www.myeloma.org

Kidney Cancer Association: www.nkca.org

Lance Armstrong Foundation: www.laf.org

The Leukemia & Lymphoma Society: www.leukemia.org

Lymphoma Research Foundation: www.lymphoma.org

Multiple Myeloma Research Foundation: www.multiplemyeloma.org

National Breast Cancer Coalition: www.natlbcc.org

National Coalition for Cancer Survivorship: www.canceradvocacy.org

National Comprehensive Cancer Network: www.nccn.org

National Lung Cancer Partnership: www.NationalLungCancerPartnership.org

National Patient Advocate Foundation: www.npaf.org

North American Brain Tumor Coalition: www.nabraintumor.org

Ovarian Cancer National Alliance: www.ovariancancer.org

Pancreatic Cancer Action Network: www.pancan.org

Prevent Cancer Foundation: www.preventcancer.org

Sarcoma Foundation of America: www.curesarcoma.org

Susan G. Komen for the Cure Advocacy Alliance: www.komenadvocacy.org

U.S. TOO International Prostate Cancer Education and Support Network: www.ustoo.com

The Wellness Community: www.thewellnesscommunity.org

The text describes in more detail how a personal health record (PHR) can help you focus your care after treatment has completed.

Many PHRs now exist using a similar template. This version for a variety of cancers stresses what *you* need to do after treatment, more than a catalog of treatment you have received.

Treatments change over time, so it is possible that the chemotherapy or type of radiation therapy listed does not match yours. Please personalize these forms on the following pages so that they remain current and meaningful to you.

The American Society of Clinical Oncology's patient resource site (http://www.cancer.net) has a selection of specialized forms using the same format. Journey Forward (http://www.journeyforward.org) has similar documents available through its website. LiveStrong—The Lance Armstrong Foundation (http://www.livestrong.org) has funded seminal programs in this area. New formats will continually be improved and available.

To Use Your Personal Health Record

Each PHR has two pages. Page 1 is tailored to many specific cancers. If your type is not listed, use the "General template". Page 2 applies to each type of cancer listed. Please be sure to copy **both pages** for each PHR.

PHR forms

PERSONAL HEALTH RECORD

Last Name: First Name:
DOB: Age: Gender: Date:
Day Phone: Evening Phone:
Address: City: State: Zip:
Email:
My Insurance: Policy #:

Spouse/Relative/Caretaker: Phone:
Health Care Proxy: Phone:

MEDICAL INFORMATION

Type of Cancer: Date of diagnosis:
Staging T: N: M:

My Health Care Team   **Phone:**   **Email:**
Medical Oncologist:
Radiation Oncologist:
Surgeon:
Fellow:
Nurse Practitioner:
Integrative Oncology Nurse:
Speech/Swallowing Therapist:
Pain/Symptom Management:
Dentist/Orthodontist:
Nutritionist:
Physical Therapist:
Social Worker:

Treatments received:
Surgical Procedures:

Chemotherapy: ☐ (mg) ☐ (mg) ☐ (mg)
☐ (mg) ☐ (mg) ☐ other
Freq: Total Dose:

Radiation Therapy:
Area treated:
☐ External Beam Radiation Therapy (EBRT)   Last Date: Dose:
☐ Brachytherapy   Last Date: Procedure: Dose:

FOLLOW-UP APPOINTMENTS:

Follow-ups: *Remember to follow up with your providers on a regular schedule*

☐ Surgical: ☐ Radiation Oncology: ☐ Medical Oncology:
☐ Cancer Supportive Services: ☐ Pain/Symptom Management: ☐ Nutrition:
☐ Speech/Swallowing Therapy: ☐ Physical Therapy: ☐ Social Work:
☐ Dental:

IMPORTANT FOLLOW-UP CARE:

Physical Therapy: *Practice the exercises you have been given by our staff to manage the following*   **Contact:** _____

☐ Secretions ☐ Pain ☐ Fatigue ☐ Neck Mobility

Nutritional Management: *See your nutritionist within 1 month post treatment to develop a plan for optimal nutrition and to manage symptoms*   **Contact:** _____

Height: Current Weight: Ideal Body Weight: Weight History:
PEG placed: PEG removed: Formula:
Recommendations:
Eating orally? ☐ Yes ☐ No   - Weaning from a PEG is a process and it can't be done immediately
                             - Food progression is gradual
Texture tolerance:
Follow up with the Nutritionist to address ongoing concerns related to nutrition, weight status and eating including any of the following symptoms:
☐ Chewing ☐ Sore throat
☐ Dry/sensitive mouth ☐ Mouth sores
☐ Changes in taste

Treatment-Related Medications: *Remember to take your medicines as scheduled*

Exams: *Do the appropriate exams as scheduled*
Blood tests: Thyroid function:

Scans:
X-ray: PET/CT: CT: Other:
Self exams:

Integrative Oncology: *Follow up as needed* Contact: _____

☐ Acupuncture
Breath/relaxation techniques: ☐ Guided imagery ☐ Progressive relaxation ☐ Autogenics
Energy therapy: ☐ Reiki ☐ Therapeutic Touch ☐ Acupressure

Speech and Swallowing: *Practice what you have been taught by our staff*
Contact: _____

- Follow up with your speech and swallowing therapist after completing treatment
- If you had surgery, get a baseline swallowing test after your surgeon clears you for eating orally
Speech Evaluation: ☐ Yes ☐ No
Results:
Swallowing Evaluation: ☐ Yes ☐ No
Results:
Acceptable diet choices:
☐ Thin Liquids ☐ Thick liquids ☐ Purees
☐ Soft Solids ☐ Unrestricted diet

Dental Care: *See your dentist for routine checkups* Contact: _____
- Teeth/gums care: thoroughly brush your teeth; floss carefully and avoid gum irritation
- Fluoride regimen: apply fluoride in a prescribed manner
- Other oral care:

Breathing: *Practice what you have been taught by our staff*
☐ Stoma care

Other:

ADJUSTING TO SURVIVORSHIP

Contact your social worker if you are experiencing distress
in any of the following areas Contact: _____

☐ Body-image ☐ Eating/sleeping patterns ☐ Disinterest in activities that you enjoy
☐ Pervasive concerns and worry ☐ Relationships with your family and friends ☐ Relationship with partner
☐ Changes in mood ☐ Sadness ☐ Fears
☐ Nervousness

WELLNESS

Avoid: Maintain:
☐ Nicotine and Tobacco Products ☐ Healthy nutrition
☐ Alcohol use ☐ Physical activity
☐ Drug use ☐ Screening for other cancers
☐ Overexposure to the sun

Screening for other cancers:
☐ Colonoscopy ☐ Mammogram ☐ PSA/Digital Rectal exam ☐ PAP/HPV tests ☐ Skin exam

ADDITIONAL INFORMATION

Organizations/Programs:	Contact Info:	Website:
Alcoholics Anonymous (AA)	Many local groups exist	http://www.alcoholics-anonymous.org
Narcotics Anonymous (NA)	Many local groups exist	http://www.na.org

Cancer Support Groups:	Contact Info:	Website:
American Cancer Society	1-800-ACS-2345	http://www.cancer.org
CancerCare	1-800-813-HOPE	http://www.cancercare.org
People Living With Cancer		http://www.cancer.net
National Cancer Institute (NCI)	1-800-4-CANCER	http://www.cancer.gov
NCI Office of Cancer Survivorship	1-301-402-2964	http://dccps.nci.nih.gov/ocs
Gilda's Club	1-888-GILDA-4-U	http://www.gildasclubnyc.org
LIVESTRONG	1-866-235-7205	http://www.livestrong.org

PERSONAL HEALTH RECORD
BRAIN OR SPINAL CORD CANCER

Last Name: First Name:
DOB: Age: Gender: Date:
Day Phone: Evening Phone:
Address: City: State: Zip:
Email:
My Insurance: Policy #:

Spouse/Relative/Caretaker: Phone:
Health Care Agent: Phone:

MEDICAL INFORMATION

Cell type: Topography (location)   Date of diagnosis:
WHO Classification

My Health Care Team   **Phone:**   **Email:**
Medical Oncologist:
Radiation Oncologist:
Surgeon:
Fellow:
Nurse Practitioner:
Integrative Oncology Nurse:
Speech/Swallowing Therapist:
Pain/Symptom Management:
Dentist/Orthodontist:
Nutritionist:
Physical Therapist:
Social Worker:

Treatments received:
Surgical Procedures:

Chemotherapy: ☐ temozolomide (mg)   ☐ CCNU (mg)   ☐ procarbazine (mg)
☐ vincristine (mg)   ☐ bevacizumab (mg)   ☐ other
Freq: Total Doses:

Radiation Therapy:
Area treated:
☐ External Beam Radiation Therapy   Last Date: Dose:
(EBRT)
☐ Stereotactic Radiosurgery   Date: Procedure: Dose:

FOLLOW-UP APPOINTMENTS:
Follow-ups: *Remember to follow up with your providers on a regular schedule*

☐ Surgical: ☐ Radiation Oncology: ☐ Medical Oncology:
☐ Cancer Supportive Services:
                             ☐ Pain/Symptom Management: ☐ Nutrition:
☐ Speech/Swallowing Therapy:
                             ☐ Physical Therapy: ☐ Social Work:
☐ Dental:

IMPORTANT FOLLOW-UP CARE:

Physical Therapy: *Practice the exercises you have been given by our
staff to manage the following*   **Contact:** _____

☐ Movement or   ☐ Cognitive impairment
Strength   ☐ Pain   ☐ Fatigue

Nutritional Management: *See your nutritionist within 1 month post
treatment to develop a plan for optimal nutrition and to manage symptoms*   **Contact:** _____

Height: Current Weight: Ideal Body Weight: Weight History:
PEG placed: PEG removed: Formula:
                     Recommendations:
Eating orally? ☐ Yes ☐ No   - Weaning from a PEG is a <u>process</u> and it <u>can't be done immediately</u>
                             - Food progression is <u>gradual</u>
Texture tolerance:
*Follow up with the Nutritionist to address ongoing concerns related to nutrition, weight status and eating including any of the
following symptoms:*
☐ Chewing   ☐ Sore throat
☐ Dry/sensitive mouth   ☐ Mouth sores
☐ Changes in taste

Treatment-Related Medications: *Remember to take your medicines as scheduled*

Exams: *Do the appropriate exams as scheduled*
Blood tests: Thyroid function:

Scans:
X-ray: PET/CT: CT: Other:
Self exams:

Integrative Oncology: *Follow up as needed*   **Contact:** _____

☐ Acupuncture
Breath/relaxation techniques: ☐ Guided imagery   ☐ Progressive relaxation   ☐ Autogenics
Energy therapy: ☐ Reiki   ☐ Therapeutic Touch   ☐ Acupressure

Speech and Swallowing: *Practice what you have been taught by our staff*
                                                                   Contact: _____

- *Follow up with your speech and swallowing therapist after completing treatment*
- *If you had surgery, get a baseline swallowing test after your surgeon clears you for eating orally*
Speech Evaluation: ☐ Yes ☐ No
Results:
Swallowing Evaluation: ☐ Yes ☐ No
Results:
Acceptable diet choices:
☐ Thin Liquids   ☐ Thick liquids   ☐ Purees
☐ Soft Solids   ☐ Unrestricted diet

Dental Care: *See your dentist for routine checkups*   **Contact:** _____
   ▪   Teeth/gums care: thoroughly brush your teeth; floss carefully and avoid gum irritation
   ▪   Fluoride regimen: apply fluoride in a prescribed manner
   ▪   Other oral care:

Breathing: *Practice what you have been taught by our staff*
☐ Stoma care

Other:

ADJUSTING TO SURVIVORSHIP

Contact your social worker if you are experiencing distress
in any of the following areas   **Contact:** _____

☐ Body-image   ☐ Eating/sleeping patterns   ☐ Disinterest in activities that you enjoy
                                ☐ Relationships with your family
☐ Pervasive concerns and worry and friends   ☐ Relationship with partner
☐ Changes in mood   ☐ Sadness   ☐ Fears
☐ Nervousness

WELLNESS

Avoid: **Maintain:**
☐ Nicotine and Tobacco Products   ☐ Healthy nutrition
☐ Alcohol use   ☐ Physical activity
☐ Drug use   ☐ Screening for other cancers
☐ Overexposure to the sun

Screening for other cancers:
☐ Colonoscopy   ☐ Mammogram   ☐ PSA/Digital Rectal exam   ☐ PAP/HPV tests   ☐ Skin exam

ADDITIONAL INFORMATION

Organizations/Programs:	Contact Info:	Website:
Alcoholics Anonymous (AA)	Many local groups exist	http://www.alcoholics-anonymous.org
Narcotics Anonymous (NA)	Many local groups exist	http://www.na.org

Cancer Support Groups:	Contact Info:	Website:
American Cancer Society	1-800-ACS-2345	http://www.cancer.org
Cancer*Care*	1-800-813-HOPE	http://www.cancercare.org
People Living With Cancer		http://www.cancer.net
National Cancer Institute (NCI)	1-800-4-CANCER	http://www.cancer.gov
NCI Office of Cancer Survivorship	1-301-402-2964	http://dccps.nci.nih.gov/ocs
Gilda's Club	1-888-GILDA-4-U	http://www.gildasclubnyc.org
LIVESTRONG	1-866-235-7205	http://www.livestrong.org

172

PERSONAL HEALTH RECORD
BREAST CANCER

Last Name: First Name:
DOB: Age: Gender: Date:
Day Phone: Evening Phone:
Address: City: State: Zip:
Email:
My Insurance: Policy #:

Spouse/Relative/Caretaker: Phone:
Health Care Agent: Phone:

MEDICAL INFORMATION

Type of Breast Cancer: Date of diagnosis:
Staging   T: N: M:

My Health Care Team   **Phone:**   **Email:**
Medical Oncologist:
Radiation Oncologist:
Surgeon:
Fellow:
Gynecologist
Nurse/Nurse Practitioner:
Integrative Oncology Nurse:
Lymphedema Specialist:
Pain/Symptom Management:
Social Worker:
Nutritionist:
Physical Therapist:
Patient Navigator:

Treatments received:
Surgical Procedures:

Chemotherapy: ☐ adriamycin   (mg)   ☐ cyclophosphamide   (mg)   ☐ pactitaxel   (mg)
☐ 5-FU   (mg)   ☐ Herceptin   (mg)   ☐ other
Freq: Total Dose:
Hormonal Treatments: ☐Arimidex ☐tamoxifen ☐ Femara (letrozole)
Radiation Therapy:
Area treated:
☐ External Beam Radiation Therapy
(EBRT)   Last Date: Dose:
☐ Brachytherapy   Last Date: Procedure: Dose:

FOLLOW-UP APPOINTMENTS:
Follow-ups: *Remember to follow up with your providers on a regular schedule*

☐ Surgical: ☐ Radiation Oncology: ☐ Medical Oncology:
☐ Cancer Supportive Services: ☐ Pain/Symptom Management: ☐ Nutrition:
☐ Gynecological   ☐ Physical Therapy: ☐ Social Work:

IMPORTANT FOLLOW-UP CARE:
Hot Flashes: number per day   interferes with comfort or functioning
Cognitive Impairment ("chemobrain")
Physical Therapy: *Practice the exercises you have been given by our*   **Contact:** _____
staff to manage the following
☐ Swelling of Arm   ☐ Pain ☐ Weight Gain   ☐ Fatigue   ☐ Range of Motion

Nutritional Management: *See your nutritionist within 1 month post*
treatment to develop a plan for optimal nutrition and to manage symptoms **Contact:** _____

Height: Current Weight: Ideal Body Weight: Weight History:
Weight gain or loss:

Follow up with the Nutritionist to address ongoing concerns related to nutrition, weight status and eating including any of the
following symptoms:
☐ Relying on comfort foods   ☐ Changes in taste
☐ Dry/sensitive mouth   ☐ Mouth sores
☐ Changes in taste

Treatment-Related Medications: *Remember to take your medicines as scheduled*

Exams: *Do the appropriate exams as scheduled*
Blood tests: Thyroid function:

Scans:
X-ray: PET/CT: CT: Other:
Self exams:

Integrative Oncology: *Follow up as needed*   **Contact:** _____

☐ Acupuncture
Breath/relaxation techniques: ☐ Guided imagery   ☐ Progressive relaxation   ☐ Autogenics
Energy therapy: ☐ Reiki   ☐ Therapeutic Touch   ☐ Acupressure

---

Speech and Swallowing: *Practice what you have been taught by our staff*
                                                        Contact: _____

- Follow up with your speech and swallowing therapist after completing treatment
- If you had surgery, get a baseline swallowing test after your surgeon clears you for eating orally
Speech Evaluation: ☐ Yes ☐ No
Results:
Swallowing Evaluation: ☐ Yes ☐ No
Results:
Acceptable diet choices:
☐ Thin Liquids   ☐ Thick liquids   ☐ Purees
☐ Soft Solids   ☐ Unrestricted diet

Dental Care: *See your dentist for routine checkups*   **Contact:** _____
- Teeth/gums care: thoroughly brush your teeth; floss carefully and avoid gum irritation
- Fluoride regimen: apply fluoride if advised
- Other oral care:

Breathing: *Practice what you have been taught by our staff*
☐

Other:

ADJUSTING TO SURVIVORSHIP

Contact your social worker if you are experiencing distress
in any of the following areas   **Contact:** _____

☐ Body-image   ☐ Eating/sleeping patterns   ☐ Disinterest in activities that you enjoy
☐ Pervasive concerns and worry   ☐ Relationships with your family   ☐ Relationship with partner
                          and friends
☐ Changes in mood   ☐ Sadness   ☐ Fears
☐ Nervousness

WELLNESS

Avoid: **Maintain:**
☐ Nicotine and Tobacco Products   ☐ Healthy nutrition
☐ Alcohol use   ☐ Physical activity
☐ Drug use   ☐ Screening for other cancers
☐ Overexposure to the sun

Screening for other cancers:
☐ Colonoscopy   ☐ Mammogram   ☐ PSA/Digital Rectal exam   ☐ PAP/HPV tests   ☐ Skin exam

---

ADDITIONAL INFORMATION

Organizations/Programs:	Contact Info:	Website:
Alcoholics Anonymous (AA)	Many local groups exist	http://www.alcoholics-anonymous.org
Narcotics Anonymous (NA)	Many local groups exist	http://www.na.org

Cancer Support Groups:	Contact Info:	Website:
American Cancer Society	1-800-ACS-2345	http://www.cancer.org
Cancer*Care*	1-800-813-HOPE	http://www.cancercare.org
People Living With Cancer		http://www.cancer.net
National Cancer Institute (NCI)	1-800-4-CANCER	http://www.cancer.gov
NCI Office of Cancer Survivorship	1-301-402-2964	http://dccps.nci.nih.gov/ocs
Gilda's Club	1-888-GILDA-4-U	http://www.gildasclubnyc.org
LIVESTRONG	1-866-235-7205	http://www.livestrong.org

PERSONAL HEALTH RECORD
COLORECTAL OR GASTRIC CANCER

Last Name: First Name:
DOB: Age: Gender: Date:
Day Phone: Evening Phone:
Address: City: State: Zip:
Email:
My Insurance: Policy #:

Spouse/Relative/Caretaker: Phone:
Health Care Agent: Phone:

MEDICAL INFORMATION

Type of cancer: Date of diagnosis:
Staging   T: N: M:

My Health Care Team   **Phone:**   **Email:**
Medical Oncologist:
Radiation Oncologist:
GI Surgeon:
Fellow:
Gastroenterologist:
Nurse/Nurse Practitioner:
Integrative Oncology Nurse:
Pain/Symptom Management:
Social Worker:
Nutritionist:
Physical Therapist:
Patient Navigator:
Enterostomal Therapist:
Treatments received:
Surgical Procedures:

Chemotherapy: ☐ 5-FU   (mg)   ☐ oxaliplatin   (mg)   ☐ Avastin   (mg)
☐ capecitabine   ☐ leucovorin   (mg)   ☐ other
(mg)
Freq: Total Dose:
Hormonal Treatments: ☐ ☐ ☐
Radiation Therapy:
Area treated:
☐ External Beam Radiation Therapy   Last Date: Dose:
(EBRT)
☐ Brachytherapy   Last Date: Procedure: Dose:

FOLLOW-UP APPOINTMENTS:
Follow-ups: _Remember to follow up with your providers on a regular schedule_

☐ Surgical: ☐ Radiation Oncology: ☐ Medical Oncology:
☐ Cancer Supportive Services: ☐ Pain/Symptom Management: ☐ Nutrition:
☐ Gastroenterologist   ☐ Physical Therapy: ☐ Social Work:

IMPORTANT FOLLOW-UP CARE:
Shortness of Breath   Blood when: number per day
Taper and avoid nicotine products   Avoid alcoholic beverages
Physical Therapy: _Practice the exercises you have been given by our_   **Contact:** _____
staff to manage the following
☐ Trouble urinating   ☐ Pain when urinating   ☐ Pain in pelvis   ☐ Fatigue

---

Nutritional Management: _See your nutritionist within 1 month post_
treatment to develop a plan for optimal nutrition and to manage symptoms   **Contact:** _____

Height: Current Weight: Ideal Body Weight: Weight History:
Weight gain or loss:

Follow up with the Nutritionist to address ongoing concerns related to nutrition, weight status and eating including any of the
following symptoms:
☐ Relying on comfort foods   ☐ Breathing exercise; rehabilitation
☐ Dry/sensitive mouth   ☐ Mouth sores
☐ Changes in taste

Treatment-Related Medications: *Remember to take your medicines as scheduled*

Exams: *Do the appropriate exams as scheduled*
Blood tests: Thyroid function:

Scans:
X-ray: PET/CT: CT: Other:
Self exams:

Integrative Oncology: *Follow up as needed*   **Contact:** _____

☐ Acupuncture
Breath/relaxation techniques: ☐ Guided imagery   ☐ Progressive relaxation   ☐ Autogenics
Energy therapy: ☐ Reiki   ☐ Therapeutic Touch   ☐ Acupressure

Speech and Swallowing: *Practice what you have been taught by our staff*   **Contact:** _____

- *Follow up with your speech and swallowing therapist after completing treatment*
- *If you had surgery, get a baseline swallowing test after your surgeon clears you for eating orally*
Speech Evaluation: ☐ Yes ☐ No
Results:
Swallowing Evaluation: ☐ Yes ☐ No
Results:
Acceptable diet choices:
☐ Thin Liquids   ☐ Thick liquids   ☐ Purees
☐ Soft Solids   ☐ Unrestricted diet

Dental Care: *See your dentist for routine checkups*   **Contact:** _____
- Teeth/gums care: thoroughly brush your teeth; floss carefully and avoid gum irritation
- Fluoride regimen: apply fluoride if advised
- Other oral care:

Breathing: *Practice what you have been taught by our staff*
☐ Stoma care

Other:

ADJUSTING TO SURVIVORSHIP

*Contact your social worker if you are experiencing distress
in any of the following areas*   **Contact:** _____

☐ Body-image   ☐ Eating/sleeping patterns   ☐ Disinterest in activities that you enjoy
                             ☐ Relationships with your family
☐ Pervasive concerns and worry   and friends   ☐ Relationship with partner

☐ Changes in mood   ☐ Sadness   ☐ Fears
☐ Nervousness

WELLNESS

Avoid: **Maintain:**
☐ Nicotine and Tobacco Products   ☐ Healthy nutrition
☐ Alcohol use   ☐ Physical activity
☐ Drug use   ☐ Screening for other cancers
☐ Overexposure to the sun

Screening for other cancers:
☐ Colonoscopy   ☐ Mammogram   ☐ PSA/Digital Rectal exam   ☐ PAP/HPV tests   ☐ Skin exam

ADDITIONAL INFORMATION

Organizations/Programs:	Contact Info:	Website:
Alcoholics Anonymous (AA)	Many local groups exist	http://www.alcoholics-anonymous.org
Narcotics Anonymous (NA)	Many local groups exist	http://www.na.org

Cancer Support Groups:	Contact Info:	Website:
American Cancer Society	1-800-ACS-2345	http://www.cancer.org
Cancer*Care*	1-800-813-HOPE	http://www.cancercare.org
People Living With Cancer		http://www.cancer.net
National Cancer Institute (NCI)	1-800-4-CANCER	http://www.cancer.gov
NCI Office of Cancer Survivorship	1-301-402-2964	http://dccps.nci.nih.gov/ocs
Gilda's Club	1-888-GILDA-4-U	http://www.gildasclubnyc.org
LIVESTRONG	1-866-235-7205	http://www.livestrong.org

PERSONAL HEALTH RECORD
GYNECOLOGIC CANCER

Last Name: First Name:
DOB: Age: Gender: Date:
Day Phone: Evening Phone:
Address: City: State: Zip:
Email:
My Insurance: Policy #:

Spouse/Relative/Caretaker: Phone:
Health Care Agent: Phone:

MEDICAL INFORMATION

Type of cancer: Date of diagnosis:
Staging   T: N: M:

My Health Care Team   **Phone:**   **Email:**
Medical Oncologist:
Radiation Oncologist:
GI Surgeon:
Fellow:
Gynecologist:
Nurse/Nurse Practitioner:
Integrative Oncology Nurse:
Pain/Symptom Management:
Social Worker:
Nutritionist:
Physical Therapist:
Patient Navigator:
Enterostomal Therapist:
Treatments received:
Surgical Procedures:

Chemotherapy: ☐ carboplatinum   ☐ paclitaxel   (mg)   ☐ PEG-adriamycin
                   (mg)   (mg)
☐   (mg)   ☐   (mg)   ☐ other
Freq: Total Dose:
Hormonal Treatments: ☐ ☐ ☐
Radiation Therapy:
Area treated:
☐ External Beam Radiation Therapy   Last Date: Dose:
(EBRT)
☐ Brachytherapy   Last Date: Procedure: Dose:

FOLLOW-UP APPOINTMENTS:
Follow-ups: *Remember to follow up with your providers on a regular schedule*

☐ Surgical: ☐ Radiation Oncology: ☐ Medical Oncology:
☐ Cancer Supportive Services: ☐ Pain/Symptom Management: ☐ Nutrition:

☐ Gastroenterologist   ☐ Physical Therapy: ☐ Social Work:

IMPORTANT FOLLOW-UP CARE:
Shortness of Breath   Blood when: number per day
Taper and avoid nicotine products   Avoid alcoholic beverages
Physical Therapy: *Practice the exercises you have been given by our*
staff to manage the following   **Contact:** _____
☐ Trouble urinating   ☐ Pain when urinating   ☐ Pain in pelvis   ☐ Fatigue

Nutritional Management: *See your nutritionist within 1 month post*
treatment to develop a plan for optimal nutrition and to manage symptoms **Contact:** _____

Height: Current Weight: Ideal Body Weight: Weight History:
Weight gain or loss:

Follow up with the Nutritionist to address ongoing concerns related to nutrition, weight status and eating including any of the
following symptoms:
☐ Relying on comfort foods   ☐ Breathing exercise; rehabilitation
☐ Dry/sensitive mouth   ☐ Mouth sores
☐ Changes in taste

Treatment-Related Medications: *Remember to take your medicines as scheduled*

Exams: *Do the appropriate exams as scheduled*
Blood tests: Thyroid function:

Scans:
X-ray: PET/CT: CT: Other:
Self exams:

Integrative Oncology: *Follow up as needed*   **Contact:** _____

☐ Acupuncture
Breath/relaxation techniques: ☐ Guided imagery   ☐ Progressive relaxation   ☐ Autogenics
Energy therapy: ☐ Reiki   ☐ Therapeutic Touch   ☐ Acupressure

Speech and Swallowing: *Practice what you have been taught by our staff*
                                                        Contact: _____

- *Follow up with your speech and swallowing therapist after completing treatment*
- *If you had surgery, get a baseline swallowing test after your surgeon clears you for eating orally*
Speech Evaluation: ☐ Yes ☐ No
Results:
Swallowing Evaluation: ☐ Yes ☐ No
Results:
Acceptable diet choices:
☐ Thin Liquids   ☐ Thick liquids   ☐ Purees
☐ Soft Solids   ☐ Unrestricted diet

Dental Care: *See your dentist for routine checkups*   **Contact:** _____
   - Teeth/gums care: thoroughly brush your teeth; floss carefully and avoid gum irritation
   - Fluoride regimen: apply fluoride if advised
   - Other oral care:

Breathing: *Practice what you have been taught by our staff*
☐ Stoma care

Other:

ADJUSTING TO SURVIVORSHIP

Contact your social worker if you are experiencing distress
in any of the following areas   **Contact:** _____

☐ Body-image   ☐ Eating/sleeping patterns   ☐ Disinterest in activities that you enjoy

☐ Pervasive concerns and worry ☐ Relationships with your family   ☐ Relationship with partner
                                 and friends

☐ Changes in mood   ☐ Sadness   ☐ Fears
☐ Nervousness

WELLNESS

Avoid: **Maintain:**
☐ Nicotine and Tobacco Products   ☐ Healthy nutrition
☐ Alcohol use   ☐ Physical activity
☐ Drug use   ☐ Screening for other cancers
☐ Overexposure to the sun

Screening for other cancers:
☐ Colonoscopy   ☐ Mammogram   ☐ PSA/Digital Rectal exam   ☐ PAP/HPV tests   ☐ Skin exam

ADDITIONAL INFORMATION

Organizations/Programs:	**Contact Info:**	**Website:**
Alcoholics Anonymous (AA)	Many local groups exist	http://www.alcoholics-anonymous.org
Narcotics Anonymous (NA)	Many local groups exist	http://www.na.org

Cancer Support Groups:	**Contact Info:**	**Website:**
American Cancer Society	1-800-ACS-2345	http://www.cancer.org
Cancer*Care*	1-800-813-HOPE	http://www.cancercare.org
People Living With Cancer		http://www.cancer.net
National Cancer Institute (NCI)	1-800-4-CANCER	http://www.cancer.gov
NCI Office of Cancer Survivorship	1-301-402-2964	http://dccps.nci.nih.gov/ocs
Gilda's Club	1-888-GILDA-4-U	http://www.gildasclubnyc.org
LIVESTRONG	1-866-235-7205	http://www.livestrong.org

PERSONAL HEALTH RECORD
HEAD AND NECK CANCERS

Last Name: First Name:
DOB: Age: Gender: Date:
Day Phone: Evening Phone:
Address: City: State: Zip:
Email:
My Insurance: Policy #:

Spouse/Relative/Caretaker: Phone:
Health Care Agent: Phone:

MEDICAL INFORMATION

Type of Cancer: Date of diagnosis:
Staging   T: N: M:

My Health Care Team   **Phone:**   **Email:**
Medical Oncologist:
Radiation Oncologist:
Surgeon:
Fellow:
Nurse Practitioner:
Integrative Oncology Nurse:
Speech/Swallowing Therapist:
Pain/Symptom Management:
Dentist/Orthodontist:
Nutritionist:
Physical Therapist:
Social Worker:

Treatments received:
Surgical Procedures:

Chemotherapy: ☐ cisplatin   (mg) ☐ carboplatin   (mg) ☐ pactitaxel   (mg)
☐ 5-FU   (mg)   ☐ cetuximab   (mg)   ☐ other
Freq: Total Dose:

Radiation Therapy:
Area treated:
☐ External Beam Radiation Therapy (EBRT)   Last Date: Dose:
☐ Brachytherapy   Last Date: Procedure: Dose:

FOLLOW-UP APPOINTMENTS:

Follow-ups: *Remember to follow up with your providers on a regular schedule*

☐ Surgical: ☐ Radiation Oncology: ☐ Medical Oncology:
☐ Cancer Supportive Services: ☐ Pain/Symptom Management: ☐ Nutrition:

☐ Speech/Swallowing Therapy: ☐ Physical Therapy: ☐ Social Work:

☐ Dental:

IMPORTANT FOLLOW-UP CARE:

Physical Therapy: *Practice the exercises you have been given by our staff to manage the following*   **Contact:** _____

☐ Secretions   ☐ Pain   ☐ Fatigue   ☐ Neck Mobility

Nutritional Management: *See your nutritionist within 1 month post treatment to develop a plan for optimal nutrition and to manage symptoms* **Contact:** _____

Height: Current Weight: Ideal Body Weight: Weight History:
PEG placed: PEG removed: Formula:
Eating orally? ☐ Yes ☐ No
Texture tolerance:
Follow up with the Nutritionist to address ongoing concerns related to nutrition, weight status and eating including any of the following symptoms:
☐ Chewing   ☐ Sore throat
☐ Dry/sensitive mouth   ☐ Mouth sores
☐ Changes in taste

Treatment-Related Medications: *Remember to take your medicines as scheduled*

Exams: *Do the appropriate exams as scheduled*
Blood tests: Thyroid function:

Scans:
X-ray: PET/CT: CT: Other:
Self exams:

Integrative Oncology: Contact:

☐ Acupuncture
Breath/relaxation techniques: ☐ Guided imagery   ☐ Progressive relaxation   ☐ Autogenics
Energy therapy: ☐ Reiki   ☐ Therapeutic Touch   ☐ Acupressure

Speech and Swallowing: *Practice what you have been taught by our staff*
                                              Contact:

- Follow up with your speech and swallowing therapist after completing treatment
- If you had surgery, get a baseline swallowing test after your surgeon clears you for eating orally
Speech Evaluation: ☐ Yes ☐ No
Results:
Swallowing Evaluation: ☐ Yes ☐ No
Results:
Acceptable diet choices:
☐ Thin Liquids   ☐ Thick liquids   ☐ Purees
☐ Soft Solids   ☐ Unrestricted diet

Recommendations:
- Weaning from a PEG is a <u>process</u> and it <u>can't be done immediately</u>
- Food progression is <u>gradual</u>

Dental Care: *See your dentist for routine checkups*   Contact:
    •   Teeth/gums care: thoroughly brush your teeth; floss carefully and avoid gum irritation
    •   Fluoride regimen: apply fluoride in a prescribed manner
    •   Other oral care:

Breathing: *Practice what you have been taught by our staff*
☐ Stoma care

Other:

ADJUSTING TO SURVIVORSHIP

Contact your social worker if you are experiencing distress
in any of the following areas   Contact:

☐ Body-image   ☐ Eating/sleeping patterns   ☐ Disinterest in activities that you enjoy
                       ☐ Relationships with your family
☐ Pervasive concerns and worry   and friends   ☐ Relationship with partner
☐ Changes in mood   ☐ Sadness   ☐ Fears
☐ Nervousness

WELLNESS

Avoid: Maintain:
☐ Nicotine and Tobacco Products   ☐ Healthy nutrition
☐ Alcohol use   ☐ Physical activity
☐ Drug use   ☐ Screening for other cancers
☐ Overexposure to the sun

Screening for other cancers:
☐ Colonoscopy   ☐ Mammogram   ☐ PSA/Digital Rectal exam   ☐ PAP/HPV tests   ☐ Skin exam

ADDITIONAL INFORMATION

Organizations/Programs:	Contact Info:	Website:
Alcoholics Anonymous (AA)	Many local groups exist	http://www.alcoholics-anonymous.org
Narcotics Anonymous (NA)	Many local groups exist	http://www.na.org

Cancer Support Groups:	Contact Info:	Website:
American Cancer Society	1-800-ACS-2345	http://www.cancer.org
CancerCare	1-800-813-HOPE	http://www.cancercare.org
People Living With Cancer		http://www.cancer.net
National Cancer Institute (NCI)	1-800-4-CANCER	http://www.cancer.gov
NCI Office of Cancer Survivorship	1-301-402-2964	http://dccps.nci.nih.gov/ocs
Gilda's Club	1-888-GILDA-4-U	http://www.gildasclubnyc.org
LIVESTRONG	1-866-235-7205	http://www.livestrong.org

PERSONAL HEALTH RECORD
HEPATOBILIARY CANCER

Last Name: First Name:
DOB: Age: Gender: Date:
Day Phone: Evening Phone:
Address: City: State: Zip:
Email:
My Insurance: Policy #:

Spouse/Relative/Caretaker: Phone:
Health Care Agent: Phone:

MEDICAL INFORMATION

Type of cancer: Date of diagnosis:

Staging   T: N: M:

Grade: Fibrosis Score
My Health Care Team   **Phone:**   **Email:**
Medical Oncologist:
Radiation Oncologist:
GI Surgeon:
Fellow:
Gastroenterologist:
Nurse/Nurse Practitioner:
Integrative Oncology Nurse:
Pain/Symptom Management:
Social Worker:
Nutritionist:
Physical Therapist:
Patient Navigator:
Enterostomal Therapist:
Treatments received:
Surgical Procedures:

Chemotherapy: ☐ sorafenib   (mg)   ☐ 5-FU   (mg)   ☐ mitomycin   (mg)
☐ intrahepatic FUDR   ☐ Yttrium90 microspheres   ☐ other
Freq: Total Dose:

Radiation Therapy:
Area treated:
☐ External Beam Radiation Therapy   Last Date: Dose:
(EBRT)
☐ Brachytherapy   Last Date: Procedure: Dose:

FOLLOW-UP APPOINTMENTS:

Follow-ups: *Remember to follow up with your providers on a regular schedule*

☐ Surgical: ☐ Radiation Oncology: ☐ Medical Oncology:
☐ Cancer Supportive Services:
                           ☐ Pain/Symptom Management: ☐ Nutrition:
☐ Gastroenterologist   ☐ Physical Therapy: ☐ Social Work:

IMPORTANT FOLLOW-UP CARE:

Shortness of Breath   Swelling feet or abdomen   Blood tests: AFP every 3 months x 2 years, then every 6 months
Imaging: every 3-6 months x 2 years, then every year
Taper and avoid nicotine products   Avoid alcoholic beverages
Physical Therapy: *Practice the exercises you have been given by our*   **Contact:** _____
staff to manage the following
☐ range of motion   ☐ fatigue/general deconditioning   ☐ shortness of breath

Nutritional Management: *See your nutritionist within 1 month post*
treatment to develop a plan for optimal nutrition and to manage symptoms   **Contact:** _____

Height: Current Weight: Ideal Body Weight: Weight History:
Weight gain or loss:

Follow up with the Nutritionist to address ongoing concerns related to nutrition, weight status and eating including any of the
following symptoms:
☐ Relying on comfort foods   ☐ Breathing exercise; rehabilitation
☐ Dry/sensitive mouth   ☐ Mouth sores
☐ Changes in taste

Treatment-Related Medications: *Remember to take your medicines as scheduled*

Exams: *Do the appropriate exams as scheduled*
Blood tests: Thyroid function:

Scans:
X-ray: PET/CT: CT: Other:
Self exams:

Integrative Oncology: *Follow up as needed*   **Contact:** _____

☐ Acupuncture
Breath/relaxation techniques: ☐ Guided imagery   ☐ Progressive relaxation   ☐ Autogenics
Energy therapy: ☐ Reiki   ☐ Therapeutic Touch   ☐ Acupressure

Speech and Swallowing: *Practice what you have been taught by our staff*
                                                                Contact: _____

- *Follow up with your speech and swallowing therapist after completing treatment*
- *If you had surgery, get a baseline swallowing test after your surgeon clears you for eating orally*
Speech Evaluation: ☐ Yes ☐ No
Results:
Swallowing Evaluation: ☐ Yes ☐ No
Results:
Acceptable diet choices:
☐ Thin Liquids   ☐ Thick liquids   ☐ Purees
☐ Soft Solids   ☐ Unrestricted diet

Dental Care: *See your dentist for routine checkups*   **Contact:** _____
- Teeth/gums care: thoroughly brush your teeth; floss carefully and avoid gum irritation
- Fluoride regimen: apply fluoride if advised
- Other oral care:

Breathing: *Practice what you have been taught by our staff*
☐ Stoma care

Other:

ADJUSTING TO SURVIVORSHIP

*Contact your social worker if you are experiencing distress
in any of the following areas*   **Contact:** _____

☐ Body-image   ☐ Eating/sleeping patterns   ☐ Disinterest in activities that you enjoy
                              ☐ Relationships with your family
☐ Pervasive concerns and worry and friends   ☐ Relationship with partner
☐ Changes in mood   ☐ Sadness   ☐ Fears
☐ Nervousness

WELLNESS

Avoid: **Maintain:**
☐ Nicotine and Tobacco Products   ☐ Healthy nutrition
☐ Alcohol use   ☐ Physical activity
☐ Drug use   ☐ Screening for other cancers
☐ Overexposure to the sun

Screening for other cancers:
☐ Colonoscopy   ☐ Mammogram   ☐ PSA/Digital Rectal exam   ☐ PAP/HPV tests   ☐ Skin exam

ADDITIONAL INFORMATION

Organizations/Programs:	Contact Info:	Website:
Alcoholics Anonymous (AA)	Many local groups exist	http://www.alcoholics-anonymous.org
Narcotics Anonymous (NA)	Many local groups exist	http://www.na.org

Cancer Support Groups:	Contact Info:	Website:
American Cancer Society	1-800-ACS-2345	http://www.cancer.org
Cancer*Care*	1-800-813-HOPE	http://www.cancercare.org
People Living With Cancer		http://www.cancer.net
National Cancer Institute (NCI)	1-800-4-CANCER	http://www.cancer.gov
NCI Office of Cancer Survivorship	1-301-402-2964	http://dccps.nci.nih.gov/ocs
Gilda's Club	1-888-GILDA-4-U	http://www.gildasclubnyc.org
LIVESTRONG	1-866-235-7205	http://www.livestrong.org

PERSONAL HEALTH RECORD
KIDNEY OR BLADDER CANCER

Last Name: First Name:
DOB: Age: Gender: Date:
Day Phone: Evening Phone:
Address: City: State: Zip:
Email:
My Insurance: Policy #:

Spouse/Relative/Caretaker: Phone:
Health Care Agent: Phone:

MEDICAL INFORMATION

Type of Cancer: Date of diagnosis:
Staging   T: N: M:

My Health Care Team   **Phone:**   **Email:**
Medical Oncologist:
Radiation Oncologist:
Surgeon:
Fellow:
Nurse Practitioner:
Integrative Oncology Nurse:
Speech/Swallowing Therapist:
Pain/Symptom Management:
Dentist/Orthodontist:
Nutritionist:
Physical Therapist:
Social Worker:

Treatments received:
Surgical Procedures:

Chemotherapy: ☐ cisplatin   (mg)   ☐ gemcitabine   (mg)   ☐ methotrexate   (mg)
☐ paclitaxel   (mg)   ☐ doxorubicin   (mg)   ☐ other
Freq: Total Dose:
☐ sunitinib   (mg) ☐ temsirolimus   (mg) ☐ bevacizumab   (mg) ☐ pazopanib   (mg)
BCG into bladder:
Radiation Therapy:
Area treated:
☐ External Beam Radiation Therapy
(EBRT)   Last Date: Dose:
☐   Last Date: Procedure: Dose:

FOLLOW-UP APPOINTMENTS:
Follow-ups: *Remember to follow up with your providers on a regular schedule*
☐ Urine cytology or cystoscopy :   Chest, abdomen & pelvis imaging every 6 mo
Surgical: ☐ Radiation Oncology: ☐ Medical Oncology:
☐ Cancer Supportive Services:
                               ☐ Pain/Symptom Management: ☐ Nutrition:
☐ Speech/Swallowing Therapy:
                               ☐ Physical Therapy: ☐ Social Work:
☐ Dental:

IMPORTANT FOLLOW-UP CARE:
Blood work and imaging above
Physical Therapy: *Practice the exercises you have been given by our
staff to manage the following*   **Contact:** _____

☐ Secretions   ☐ Pain   ☐ Fatigue   ☐ Neck Mobility

Nutritional Management: *See your nutritionist within 1 month post
treatment to develop a plan for optimal nutrition and to manage symptoms*   **Contact:** _____

Height: Current Weight: Ideal Body Weight: Weight History:
PEG placed: PEG removed: Formula:
                     Recommendations:
Eating orally? ☐ Yes ☐ No   - Weaning from a PEG is a process and it can't be done immediately
                            - Food progression is gradual
Texture tolerance:
*Follow up with the Nutritionist to address ongoing concerns related to nutrition, weight status and eating including any of the
following symptoms:*
☐ Chewing   ☐ Sore throat
☐ Dry/sensitive mouth   ☐ Mouth sores
☐ Changes in taste

Treatment-Related Medications: *Remember to take your medicines as scheduled*

Exams: *Do the appropriate exams as scheduled*
Blood tests: Thyroid function:

Scans:
X-ray: PET/CT: CT: Other:
Self exams:

Integrative Oncology: *Follow up as needed*   Contact: _____

☐ Acupuncture
Breath/relaxation techniques: ☐ Guided imagery   ☐ Progressive relaxation   ☐ Autogenics
Energy therapy: ☐ Reiki   ☐ Therapeutic Touch   ☐ Acupressure

Speech and Swallowing: *Practice what you have been taught by our staff*   Contact: _____

- *Follow up with your speech and swallowing therapist after completing treatment*
- *If you had surgery, get a baseline swallowing test after your surgeon clears you for eating orally*
Speech Evaluation: ☐ Yes ☐ No
Results:
Swallowing Evaluation: ☐ Yes ☐ No
Results:
Acceptable diet choices:
☐ Thin Liquids   ☐ Thick liquids   ☐ Purees
☐ Soft Solids   ☐ Unrestricted diet

Dental Care: *See your dentist for routine checkups*   Contact: _____
- Teeth/gums care: thoroughly brush your teeth; floss carefully and avoid gum irritation
- Fluoride regimen: apply fluoride if advised
- Other oral care:

Breathing: *Practice what you have been taught by our staff*
☐ Stoma care

Other:

ADJUSTING TO SURVIVORSHIP

Contact your social worker if you are experiencing distress   Contact: _____
in any of the following areas
☐ Body-image   ☐ Eating/sleeping patterns   ☐ Disinterest in activities that you enjoy
☐ Pervasive concerns and worry ☐ Relationships with your family ☐ Relationship with partner
                                and friends
☐ Changes in mood   ☐ Sadness   ☐ Fears
☐ Nervousness

WELLNESS

Avoid: **Maintain:**
☐ Nicotine and Tobacco Products   ☐ Healthy nutrition
☐ Alcohol use   ☐ Physical activity
☐ Drug use   ☐ Screening for other cancers
☐ Overexposure to the sun

Screening for other cancers:
☐ Colonoscopy   ☐ Mammogram   ☐ PSA/Digital Rectal exam   ☐ PAP/HPV tests   ☐ Skin exam

ADDITIONAL INFORMATION

Organizations/Programs:	Contact Info:	Website:
Alcoholics Anonymous (AA)	Many local groups exist	http://www.alcoholics-anonymous.org
Narcotics Anonymous (NA)	Many local groups exist	http://www.na.org

Cancer Support Groups:	Contact Info:	Website:
American Cancer Society	1-800-ACS-2345	http://www.cancer.org
CancerCare	1-800-813-HOPE	http://www.cancercare.org
People Living With Cancer		http://www.cancer.net
National Cancer Institute (NCI)	1-800-4-CANCER	http://www.cancer.gov
NCI Office of Cancer Survivorship	1-301-402-2964	http://dccps.nci.nih.gov/ocs
Gilda's Club	1-888-GILDA-4-U	http://www.gildasclubnyc.org
LIVESTRONG	1-866-235-7205	http://www.livestrong.org

PERSONAL HEALTH RECORD
LEUKEMIA

Last Name: First Name:
DOB: Age: Gender: Date:
Day Phone: Evening Phone:
Address: City: State: Zip:
Email:
My Insurance: Policy #:

Spouse/Relative/Caretaker: Phone:
Health Care Agent: Phone:

MEDICAL INFORMATION

Type of Leukemia: Subtype: Stage: Date of diagnosis:

My Health Care Team   **Phone:**   **Email:**
Medical Oncologist:
Radiation Oncologist:
Surgeon:
Fellow:
Nurse Practitioner:
Integrative Oncology Nurse:
Hematologist:
Pain/Symptom Management:
Dentist/Orthodontist:
Nutritionist:
Physical Therapist:
Social Worker:

Treatments received:
Surgical Procedures:
Chemotherapy: ☐ doxorubicin   bleomycin   mg   vincistine   mg   dacarbazine   mg   rituximab   mg
                prednisone   mg   cyclophosphamide   mg ☐   (mg)   ☐ I   (mg)
☐ fludarabine   (mg)   ☐ chlorambucil   (mg)
☐ Allopurinol   (mg)   ☐ cetuximab   (mg)   ☐ rasburicase   (mg)
                           ☐ other
Freq: Total Doses:
Radiation Therapy:
Area treated:
☐ External Beam Radiation Therapy
(EBRT)   Last Date: Dose:

FOLLOW-UP APPOINTMENTS:

Follow-ups: *Remember to follow up with your providers on a regular schedule*

☐ Surgical: ☐ Radiation Oncology: ☐ Medical Oncology:
☐ Cancer Supportive Services:
                               ☐ Pain/Symptom Management: ☐ Nutrition:
☐ Speech/Swallowing Therapy:
                               ☐ Physical Therapy: ☐ Social Work:
☐ Dental:

IMPORTANT FOLLOW-UP CARE:

Physical Therapy: *Practice the exercises you have been given by our*   **Contact:** _____
staff to manage the following
☐ Fatigue/general   ☐ Shortness of breath ☐ Pain ☐ Fatigue

Nutritional Management: *See your nutritionist within 1 month post*
treatment to develop a plan for optimal nutrition and to manage symptoms   **Contact:** _____

Height: Current Weight: Ideal Body Weight: Weight History:
PEG placed: PEG removed: Formula:
                    Recommendations:
Eating orally? ☐ Yes ☐ No   - Weaning from a PEG is a process and it can't be done immediately
                             - Food progression is gradual
Texture tolerance:
Follow up with the Nutritionist to address ongoing concerns related to nutrition, weight status and eating including any of the
following symptoms:
☐ Chewing   ☐ Sore throat
☐ Dry/sensitive mouth   ☐ Mouth sores
☐ Changes in taste

Treatment-Related Medications: *Remember to take your medicines as scheduled*

Exams: *Do the appropriate exams as scheduled*
Blood tests: Thyroid function:

Scans:
X-ray: PET/CT: CT: Other:
Self exams:

Integrative Oncology: *Follow up as needed*   **Contact:** _____

☐ Acupuncture
Breath/relaxation techniques: ☐ Guided imagery   ☐ Progressive relaxation   ☐ Autogenics
Energy therapy: ☐ Reiki   ☐ Therapeutic Touch   ☐ Acupressure

Speech and Swallowing: *Practice what you have been taught by our staff*   **Contact:** _____

- *Follow up with your speech and swallowing therapist after completing treatment*
- *If you had surgery, get a baseline swallowing test after your surgeon clears you for eating orally*
Speech Evaluation: ☐ Yes ☐ No
Results:
Swallowing Evaluation: ☐ Yes ☐ No
Results:
Acceptable diet choices:
☐ Thin Liquids   ☐ Thick liquids   ☐ Purees
☐ Soft Solids   ☐ Unrestricted diet

Dental Care: *See your dentist for routine checkups*   **Contact:** _____
- Teeth/gums care: thoroughly brush your teeth; floss carefully and avoid gum irritation
- Fluoride regimen: apply fluoride if advised
- Other oral care:

Breathing: *Practice what you have been taught by our staff*
☐

Other:

ADJUSTING TO SURVIVORSHIP

*Contact your social worker if you are experiencing distress
in any of the following areas*   **Contact:** _____

☐ Body-image   ☐ Eating/sleeping patterns   ☐ Disinterest in activities that you enjoy
☐ Pervasive concerns and worry ☐ Relationships with your family   ☐ Relationship with partner
                                and friends
☐ Changes in mood   ☐ Sadness   ☐ Fears
☐ Nervousness

WELLNESS

Avoid: **Maintain:**
☐ Nicotine and Tobacco Products   ☐ Healthy nutrition
☐ Alcohol use   ☐ Physical activity
☐ Drug use   ☐ Screening for other cancers
☐ Overexposure to the sun

Screening for other cancers:
☐ Colonoscopy   ☐ Mammogram   ☐ PSA/Digital Rectal exam   ☐ PAP/HPV tests   ☐ Skin exam

ADDITIONAL INFORMATION

Organizations/Programs:	**Contact Info:**	**Website:**
Alcoholics Anonymous (AA)	Many local groups exist	http://www.alcoholics-anonymous.org
Narcotics Anonymous (NA)	Many local groups exist	http://www.na.org

Cancer Support Groups:	**Contact Info:**	**Website:**
American Cancer Society	1-800-ACS-2345	http://www.cancer.org
Cancer*Care*	1-800-813-HOPE	http://www.cancercare.org
People Living With Cancer		http://www.cancer.net
National Cancer Institute (NCI)	1-800-4-CANCER	http://www.cancer.gov
NCI Office of Cancer Survivorship	1-301-402-2964	http://dccps.nci.nih.gov/ocs
Gilda's Club	1-888-GILDA-4-U	http://www.gildasclubnyc.org
LIVESTRONG	1-866-235-7205	http://www.livestrong.org

PERSONAL HEALTH RECORD
LUNG CANCER

Last Name: First Name:
DOB: Age: Gender: Date:
Day Phone: Evening Phone:
Address: City: State: Zip:
Email:
My Insurance: Policy #:

Spouse/Relative/Caretaker: Phone:
Health Care Agent: Phone:

MEDICAL INFORMATION

Type of cancer: Date of diagnosis:
Staging   T: N: M:

My Health Care Team   **Phone:**   **Email:**
Medical Oncologist:
Radiation Oncologist:
Thoracic Surgeon:
Fellow:
Pulmonologist:
Nurse/Nurse Practitioner:
Integrative Oncology Nurse:
Pain/Symptom Management:
Social Worker:
Nutritionist:
Physical Therapist:
Patient Navigator:

Treatments received:
Surgical Procedures:

Chemotherapy: ☐ carboplatin   (mg) ☐ paclitaxel   (mg)   ☐ Avastin   (mg)
☐ Alimpta   (mg)   ☐ cisplatin   (mg) ☐ other
Freq: Total Dose:
Hormonal Treatments: ☐
Radiation Therapy:
Area treated:
☐ External Beam Radiation Therapy
(EBRT)   Last Date: Dose:
☐ Brachytherapy   Last Date: Procedure: Dose:

FOLLOW-UP APPOINTMENTS:
Follow-ups: *Remember to follow up with your providers on a regular schedule*

☐ Surgical: ☐ Radiation Oncology: ☐ Medical Oncology:
☐ Cancer Supportive Services: ☐ Pain/Symptom Management: ☐ Nutrition:

☐ Pulmonologist   ☐ Physical Therapy: ☐ Social Work:

IMPORTANT FOLLOW-UP CARE:
Shortness of Breath   Blood whens: number per day
Taper and avoid nicotine products   Avoid alcoholic beverages
Physical Therapy: *Practice the exercises you have been given by our*   Contact: _____
staff to manage the following
☐ Trouble urinating   ☐ Pain when urinating   ☐ Pain in pelvis   ☐ Fatigue

Nutritional Management: *See your nutritionist within 1 month post*
treatment to develop a plan for optimal nutrition and to manage symptoms **Contact:** _____

Height: Current Weight: Ideal Body Weight: Weight History:
Weight gain or loss:

Follow up with the Nutritionist to address ongoing concerns related to nutrition, weight status and eating including any of the
following symptoms:
☐ Relying on comfort foods   ☐ Breathing exercise; pulmonary rehabilitation
☐ Dry/sensitive mouth   ☐ Mouth sores
☐ Changes in taste

Treatment-Related Medications: *Remember to take your medicines as scheduled*

Exams: *Do the appropriate exams as scheduled*
Blood tests: Thyroid function:

Scans:
X-ray: PET/CT: CT: Other:
Self exams:

Integrative Oncology: *Follow up as needed*   **Contact:** _____

☐ Acupuncture
Breath/relaxation techniques: ☐ Guided imagery   ☐ Progressive relaxation   ☐ Autogenics
Energy therapy: ☐ Reiki   ☐ Therapeutic Touch   ☐ Acupressure

---

Speech and Swallowing: *Practice what you have been taught by our staff*
                    Contact: _____

- Follow up with your speech and swallowing therapist after completing treatment
- If you had surgery, get a baseline swallowing test after your surgeon clears you for eating orally
Speech Evaluation: ☐ Yes ☐ No
Results:
Swallowing Evaluation: ☐ Yes ☐ No
Results:
Acceptable diet choices:
☐ Thin Liquids   ☐ Thick liquids   ☐ Purees
☐ Soft Solids   ☐ Unrestricted diet

Dental Care: *See your dentist for routine checkups*   **Contact:** _____
   ▪ Teeth/gums care: thoroughly brush your teeth; floss carefully and avoid gum irritation
   ▪ Fluoride regimen: apply fluoride if advised
   ▪ Other oral care:

Breathing: *Practice what you have been taught by our staff*
☐ Stoma care

Other:

ADJUSTING TO SURVIVORSHIP

*Contact your social worker if you are experiencing distress
in any of the following areas*   **Contact:** _____

☐ Body-image   ☐ Eating/sleeping patterns   ☐ Disinterest in activities that you enjoy
                                ☐ Relationships with your family
☐ Pervasive concerns and worry and friends   ☐ Relationship with partner
☐ Changes in mood   ☐ Sadness   ☐ Fears
☐ Nervousness

WELLNESS

Avoid: **Maintain:**
☐ Nicotine and Tobacco Products   ☐ Healthy nutrition
☐ Alcohol use   ☐ Physical activity
☐ Drug use   ☐ Screening for other cancers
☐ Overexposure to the sun

Screening for other cancers:
☐ Colonoscopy   ☐ Mammogram   ☐ PSA/Digital Rectal exam   ☐ PAP/HPV tests   ☐ Skin exam

---

ADDITIONAL INFORMATION

Organizations/Programs:	Contact Info:	Website:
Alcoholics Anonymous (AA)	Many local groups exist	http://www.alcoholics-anonymous.org
Narcotics Anonymous (NA)	Many local groups exist	http://www.na.org

Cancer Support Groups:	Contact Info:	Website:
American Cancer Society	1-800-ACS-2345	http://www.cancer.org
CancerCare	1-800-813-HOPE	http://www.cancercare.org
People Living With Cancer		http://www.cancer.net
National Cancer Institute (NCI)	1-800-4-CANCER	http://www.cancer.gov
NCI Office of Cancer Survivorship	1-301-402-2964	http://dccps.nci.nih.gov/ocs
Gilda's Club	1-888-GILDA-4-U	http://www.gildasclubnyc.org
LIVESTRONG	1-866-235-7205	http://www.livestrong.org

PERSONAL HEALTH RECORD
LYMPHOMAS

Last Name: First Name:
DOB: Age: Gender: Date:
Day Phone: Evening Phone:
Address: City: State: Zip:
Email:
My Insurance: Policy #:

Spouse/Relative/Caretaker: Phone:
Health Care Agent: Phone:

MEDICAL INFORMATION

Type of Lymphoma: Date of diagnosis:
Staging   Stage: Lymphovascular   Residual

My Health Care Team   **Phone:**   **Email:**
Medical Oncologist:
Radiation Oncologist:
Surgeon:
Fellow:
Nurse Practitioner:
Integrative Oncology Nurse:
Hematologist:
Pain/Symptom Management:
Dentist:
Nutritionist:
Physical Therapist:
Social Worker:

Treatments received:
Surgical Procedures:
Chemotherapy: ☐ doxorubicin ☐ bleomycin ___ mg ☐ vincistine ___ mg ☐ dacarbazine ___ mg
         ☐ rituximab mg ☐ prednisone mg ☐ cyclophosphamide mg ☐   (mg) ☐   (mg)
         ☐ ara C   (mg)   ☐ fludarabine   (mg) ☐ chlorambucil   (mg)
                                                     ☐ other
Freq: Total Dose:

Radiation Therapy:
Area treated:
☐ External Beam Radiation Therapy   Last Date: Dose:
(EBRT)

FOLLOW-UP APPOINTMENTS:

Follow-ups: *Remember to follow up with your providers on a regular schedule*

☐ Surgical: ☐ Radiation Oncology: ☐ Medical Oncology:
☐ Cancer Supportive Services:
                            ☐ Pain/Symptom Management: ☐ Nutrition:
☐ Speech/Swallowing Therapy:
                            ☐ Physical Therapy: ☐ Social Work:
☐ Dental:

IMPORTANT FOLLOW-UP CARE:

Physical Therapy: *Practice the exercises you have been given by our*   **Contact:** _____
staff to manage the following

☐ Shortness of breath   ☐ Pain   ☐ Fatigue   ☐

Nutritional Management: *See your nutritionist within 1 month post*
treatment to develop a plan for optimal nutrition and to manage symptoms   **Contact:** _____

Height: Current Weight: Ideal Body Weight: Weight History:
PEG placed: PEG removed: Formula:
                        Recommendations:
Eating orally? ☐ Yes ☐ No   - Weaning from a PEG is a <u>process</u> and it <u>can't be done immediately</u>
                             - Food progression is <u>gradual</u>
Texture tolerance:
Follow up with the Nutritionist to address ongoing concerns related to nutrition, weight status and eating including any of the
following symptoms:
☐ Chewing   ☐ Sore throat
☐ Dry/sensitive mouth   ☐ Mouth sores
☐ Changes in taste

Treatment-Related Medications: *Remember to take your medicines as scheduled*

Exams: *Do the appropriate exams as scheduled*
Blood tests: Thyroid function:

Scans:
X-ray: PET/CT: CT: Other:
Self exams:

Integrative Oncology: *Follow up as needed*   **Contact:** _____

☐ Acupuncture
Breath/relaxation techniques: ☐ Guided imagery   ☐ Progressive relaxation   ☐ Autogenics
Energy therapy: ☐ Reiki   ☐ Therapeutic Touch   ☐ Acupressure

Speech and Swallowing: *Practice what you have been taught by our staff*
                                                        Contact: _____

- *Follow up with your speech and swallowing therapist after completing treatment*
- *If you had surgery, get a baseline swallowing test after your surgeon clears you for eating orally*
Speech Evaluation: ☐ Yes ☐ No
Results:
Swallowing Evaluation: ☐ Yes ☐ No
Results:
Acceptable diet choices:
☐ Thin Liquids   ☐ Thick liquids   ☐ Purees
☐ Soft Solids   ☐ Unrestricted diet

Dental Care: *See your dentist for routine checkups*   **Contact:** _____
- Teeth/gums care: thoroughly brush your teeth; floss carefully and avoid gum irritation
- Fluoride regimen: apply fluoride if prescribed
- Other oral care:

Breathing: *Practice what you have been taught by our staff*
☐

Other:

ADJUSTING TO SURVIVORSHIP

*Contact your social worker if you are experiencing distress
in any of the following areas*   **Contact:** _____

☐ Body-image   ☐ Eating/sleeping patterns   ☐ Disinterest in activities that you enjoy
                              ☐ Relationships with your family
☐ Pervasive concerns and worry   and friends   ☐ Relationship with partner
☐ Changes in mood   ☐ Sadness   ☐ Fears
☐ Nervousness

WELLNESS

Avoid: **Maintain:**
☐ Nicotine and Tobacco Products   ☐ Healthy nutrition
☐ Alcohol use   ☐ Physical activity
☐ Drug use   ☐ Screening for other cancers
☐ Overexposure to the sun

Screening for other cancers:
☐ Colonoscopy   ☐ Mammogram   ☐ PSA/Digital Rectal exam   ☐ PAP/HPV tests   ☐ Skin exam

ADDITIONAL INFORMATION

Organizations/Programs:	**Contact Info:**	**Website:**
Alcoholics Anonymous (AA)	Many local groups exist	http://www.alcoholics-anonymous.org
Narcotics Anonymous (NA)	Many local groups exist	http://www.na.org

Cancer Support Groups:	**Contact Info:**	**Website:**
American Cancer Society	1-800-ACS-2345	http://www.cancer.org
CancerCare	1-800-813-HOPE	http://www.cancercare.org
People Living With Cancer		http://www.cancer.net
National Cancer Institute (NCI)	1-800-4-CANCER	http://www.cancer.gov
NCI Office of Cancer Survivorship	1-301-402-2964	http://dccps.nci.nih.gov/ocs
Gilda's Club	1-888-GILDA-4-U	http://www.gildasclubnyc.org
LIVESTRONG	1-866-235-7205	http://www.livestrong.org

PERSONAL HEALTH RECORD
MYELOMA

Last Name: First Name:
DOB: Age: Gender: Date:
Day Phone: Evening Phone:
Address: City: State: Zip:
Email:
My Insurance: Policy #:

Spouse/Relative/Caretaker: Phone:
Health Care Agent: Phone:

MEDICAL INFORMATION

Plasmacytoma: Asymptomatic: Symptomatic: Date of diagnosis:

My Health Care Team   **Phone:**   **Email:**
Medical Oncologist:
Radiation Oncologist:
Surgeon:
Fellow:
Nurse Practitioner:
Integrative Oncology Nurse:
Hematologist:
Pain/Symptom Management:
Dentist:
Nutritionist:
Physical Therapist:
Social Worker:

Treatments received:
Surgical Procedures:
Chemotherapy: ☐   (mg) ☐ I   (mg)
    ☐ bortezomib   (mg)   ☐ lenalidomide   (mg)   ☐ dexamethasone   (mg)
    ☐ melphalan (mg)   ☐ thalidomide   (mg)   ☐ vincristine   (mg)   ☐ other
Freq: Total Doses:

Radiation Therapy:
Area treated:
☐ External Beam Radiation Therapy   Last Date: Dose:
(EBRT)

FOLLOW-UP APPOINTMENTS:
Follow-ups: *Remember to follow up with your providers on a regular schedule*

☐ Surgical: ☐ Radiation Oncology: ☐ Medical Oncology:
☐ Cancer Supportive Services: ☐ Pain/Symptom Management: ☐ Nutrition:

☐ Speech/Swallowing Therapy: ☐ Physical Therapy: ☐ Social Work:

☐ Dental:

IMPORTANT FOLLOW-UP CARE:

Physical Therapy: *Practice the exercises you have been given by our staff to manage the following:*   **Contact:** _____
☐ general deconditioning/fatigue ☐ balance
☐ SPEP every   weeks   ☐ CBC for anemia   ☐ Lytes for renal func every   ☐ Bone density & ?
     avoid NSAIDs   every   weeks   weeks   bisphosphonates
                   avoid IV contrast

Nutritional Management: *See your nutritionist within 1 month post treatment to develop a plan for optimal nutrition and to manage symptoms* **Contact:** _____

Height: Current Weight: Ideal Body Weight: Weight History:
PEG placed: PEG removed: Formula:
                Recommendations:
Eating orally? ☐ Yes ☐ No   - Weaning from a PEG is a process and it can't be done immediately
                   - Food progression is gradual
Texture tolerance:
Follow up with the Nutritionist to address ongoing concerns related to nutrition, weight status and eating including any of the following symptoms:
☐ Chewing   ☐ Sore throat
☐ Dry/sensitive mouth   ☐ Mouth sores
☐ Changes in taste

Treatment-Related Medications: *Remember to take your medicines as scheduled*

Exams: *Do the appropriate exams as scheduled*
Blood tests: Thyroid function:

Scans:
X-ray: PET/CT: CT: Other:
Self exams:

Integrative Oncology: *Follow up as needed*   **Contact:** _____

☐ Acupuncture
Breath/relaxation techniques: ☐ Guided imagery   ☐ Progressive relaxation   ☐ Autogenics
Energy therapy: ☐ Reiki   ☐ Therapeutic Touch   ☐ Acupressure

Speech and Swallowing: *Practice what you have been taught by our staff*
                                                                Contact: _____

- *Follow up with your speech and swallowing therapist after completing treatment*
- *If you had surgery, get a baseline swallowing test after your surgeon clears you for eating orally*
Speech Evaluation: ☐ Yes ☐ No
Results:
Swallowing Evaluation: ☐ Yes ☐ No
Results:
Acceptable diet choices:
☐ Thin Liquids   ☐ Thick liquids   ☐ Purees
☐ Soft Solids   ☐ Unrestricted diet

Dental Care: *See your dentist for routine checkups*   **Contact:** _____
- Teeth/gums care: thoroughly brush your teeth; floss carefully and avoid gum irritation
- Fluoride regimen: apply fluoride if advised
- Other oral care:

Breathing: *Practice what you have been taught by our staff*
☐

Other:

ADJUSTING TO SURVIVORSHIP

Contact your social worker if you are experiencing distress
in any of the following areas   **Contact:** _____

☐ Body-image   ☐ Eating/sleeping patterns   ☐ Disinterest in activities that you enjoy
                                ☐ Relationships with your family
☐ Pervasive concerns and worry   and friends   ☐ Relationship with partner
☐ Changes in mood   ☐ Sadness   ☐ Fears
☐ Nervousness

WELLNESS

Avoid: **Maintain:**
☐ Nicotine and Tobacco Products   ☐ Healthy nutrition
☐ Alcohol use   ☐ Physical activity
☐ Drug use   ☐ Screening for other cancers
☐ Overexposure to the sun

Screening for other cancers:
☐ Colonoscopy   ☐ Mammogram   ☐ PSA/Digital Rectal exam   ☐ PAP/HPV tests   ☐ Skin exam

ADDITIONAL INFORMATION

Organizations/Programs:	Contact Info:	Website:
Alcoholics Anonymous (AA)	Many local groups exist	http://www.alcoholics-anonymous.org
Narcotics Anonymous (NA)	Many local groups exist	http://www.na.org

Cancer Support Groups:	Contact Info:	Website:
American Cancer Society	1-800-ACS-2345	http://www.cancer.org
Cancer*Care*	1-800-813-HOPE	http://www.cancercare.org
People Living With Cancer		http://www.cancer.net
National Cancer Institute (NCI)	1-800-4-CANCER	http://www.cancer.gov
NCI Office of Cancer Survivorship	1-301-402-2964	http://dccps.nci.nih.gov/ocs
Gilda's Club	1-888-GILDA-4-U	http://www.gildasclubnyc.org
LIVESTRONG	1-866-235-7205	http://www.livestrong.org

PERSONAL HEALTH RECORD
PANCREATIC CANCER

Last Name: First Name:
DOB: Age: Gender: Date:
Day Phone: Evening Phone:
Address: City: State: Zip:
Email:
My Insurance: Policy #:

Spouse/Relative/Caretaker: Phone:
Health Care Agent: Phone:

MEDICAL INFORMATION

Type of cancer: Date of diagnosis:
Staging   T: N: M:

My Health Care Team   **Phone:**   **Email:**
Medical Oncologist:
Radiation Oncologist:
GI Surgeon:
Fellow:
Gastroenterologist:
Nurse/Nurse Practitioner:
Integrative Oncology Nurse:
Pain/Symptom Management:
Social Worker:
Nutritionist:
Physical Therapist:
Patient Navigator:

Treatments received:
Surgical Procedures:
☐ nerve block
Chemotherapy: ☐ 5-FU   (mg)   ☐ oxaliplatin   (mg)   ☐ gemcitabine   (mg)
☐ capecitabine
(mg)   ☐ leucovorin   (mg)   ☐ other
Freq: Total Dose:
☐ pancreatic enzymes
Radiation Therapy:
Area treated:
☐ External Beam Radiation Therapy   Last Date: Dose:
(EBRT)
☐ Brachytherapy   Last Date: Procedure: Dose:

FOLLOW-UP APPOINTMENTS:
Follow-ups: *Remember to follow up with your providers on a regular schedule*

☐ Surgical: ☐ Radiation Oncology: ☐ Medical Oncology:
☐ Cancer Supportive Services: ☐ Pain/Symptom Management: ☐ Nutrition:

☐ Gastroenterologist   ☐ Physical Therapy: ☐ Social Work:

IMPORTANT FOLLOW-UP CARE:
Shortness of Breath   Blood cough up: in stool
Taper and avoid nicotine products   Avoid alcoholic beverages
Physical Therapy: *Practice the exercises you have been given by our
staff to manage the following*   **Contact:** _____
☐ Trouble urinating   ☐ Pain when urinating   ☐ Pain in pelvis   ☐ Fatigue

Nutritional Management: *See your nutritionist within 1 month post
treatment to develop a plan for optimal nutrition and to manage symptoms* **Contact:** _____

Height: Current Weight: Ideal Body Weight: Weight History:
Weight gain or loss:
Supplements

*Follow up with the Nutritionist to address ongoing concerns related to nutrition, weight status and eating including any of the
following symptoms:*
☐ Relying on comfort foods   ☐ Breathing exercise; rehabilitation
☐ Dry/sensitive mouth   ☐ Mouth sores
☐ Changes in taste

Treatment-Related Medications: *Remember to take your medicines as scheduled*

Exams: *Do the appropriate exams as scheduled*
Blood tests: Thyroid function:

Scans:
X-ray: PET/CT: CT: Other:
Self exams:

Integrative Oncology: *Follow up as needed*   **Contact:** _____

☐ Acupuncture
Breath/relaxation techniques: ☐ Guided imagery   ☐ Progressive relaxation   ☐ Autogenics
Energy therapy: ☐ Reiki   ☐ Therapeutic Touch   ☐ Acupressure

Speech and Swallowing: *Practice what you have been taught by our staff*   **Contact:** _____

- *Follow up with your speech and swallowing therapist after completing treatment*
- *If you had surgery, get a baseline swallowing test after your surgeon clears you for eating orally*
Speech Evaluation: ☐ Yes ☐ No
Results:
Swallowing Evaluation: ☐ Yes ☐ No
Results:
Acceptable diet choices:
☐ Thin Liquids   ☐ Thick liquids   ☐ Purees
☐ Soft Solids   ☐ Unrestricted diet

Dental Care: *See your dentist for routine checkups*   **Contact:** _____
- Teeth/gums care: thoroughly brush your teeth; floss carefully and avoid gum irritation
- Fluoride regimen: apply fluoride if advised
- Other oral care:

Breathing: *Practice what you have been taught by our staff*
☐

Other:

ADJUSTING TO SURVIVORSHIP

Contact your social worker if you are experiencing distress
in any of the following areas   **Contact:** _____

☐ Body-image   ☐ Eating/sleeping patterns   ☐ Disinterest in activities that you enjoy

☐ Pervasive concerns and worry   ☐ Relationships with your family   ☐ Relationship with partner
                             and friends

☐ Changes in mood   ☐ Sadness   ☐ Fears
☐ Nervousness

WELLNESS

Avoid: **Maintain:**
☐ Nicotine and Tobacco Products   ☐ Healthy nutrition
☐ Alcohol use   ☐ Physical activity
☐ Drug use   ☐ Screening for other cancers
☐ Overexposure to the sun

Screening for other cancers:
☐ Colonoscopy   ☐ Mammogram   ☐ PSA/Digital Rectal exam   ☐ PAP/HPV tests   ☐ Skin exam

ADDITIONAL INFORMATION

Organizations/Programs:	Contact Info:	Website:
Alcoholics Anonymous (AA)	Many local groups exist	http://www.alcoholics-anonymous.org
Narcotics Anonymous (NA)	Many local groups exist	http://www.na.org

Cancer Support Groups:	Contact Info:	Website:
American Cancer Society	1-800-ACS-2345	http://www.cancer.org
CancerCare	1-800-813-HOPE	http://www.cancercare.org
People Living With Cancer		http://www.cancer.net
National Cancer Institute (NCI)	1-800-4-CANCER	http://www.cancer.gov
NCI Office of Cancer Survivorship	1-301-402-2964	http://dccps.nci.nih.gov/ocs
Gilda's Club	1-888-GILDA-4-U	http://www.gildasclubnyc.org
LIVESTRONG	1-866-235-7205	http://www.livestrong.org

PERSONAL HEALTH RECORD
PROSTATE CANCER

Last Name: First Name:
DOB: Age: Gender: Date:
Day Phone: Evening Phone:
Address: City: State: Zip:
Email:
My Insurance: Policy #:

Spouse/Relative/Caretaker: Phone:
Health Care Agent: Phone:

MEDICAL INFORMATION

Gleason Score: PSA=   Date of diagnosis:
Staging   T: N: M:

My Health Care Team   **Phone:**   **Email:**
Medical Oncologist:
Radiation Oncologist:
Urological Surgeon:
Fellow:
General Urologist:
Nurse/Nurse Practitioner:
Integrative Oncology Nurse:
Pain/Symptom Management:
Social Worker:
Nutritionist:
Physical Therapist:
Patient Navigator:

Treatments received:
Surgical Procedures:

Chemotherapy: ☐ corticosteorids   ☐ paclitaxel   (mg)   ☐ mitoxantrone (mg)
               (mg)
☐ paclitaxel   (mg)   ☐   (mg)   ☐ other
Freq: Total Dose:
Hormonal Treatments: ☐ Eulexin ☐Casodex ☐ Zoladex ☐ other
Radiation Therapy:
Area treated:
☐ External Beam Radiation Therapy
(EBRT)   Last Date: Dose:
☐ Brachytherapy   Last Date: Procedure: Dose:

FOLLOW-UP APPOINTMENTS:
Follow-ups: *Remember to follow up with your providers on a regular schedule*

☐ Surgical: ☐ Radiation Oncology: ☐ Medical Oncology:
☐ Cancer Supportive Services: ☐ Pain/Symptom Management: ☐ Nutrition:

☐ General Urologist   ☐ Physical Therapy: ☐ Social Work:

IMPORTANT FOLLOW-UP CARE:
Hot Flashes: number per day   interferes with comfort or functioning
Cognitive Impairment ("chemobrain")
Physical Therapy: *Practice the exercises you have been given by our staff to manage the following*   **Contact:** _____
☐ Trouble urinating   ☐ Pain when urinating   ☐ Pain in pelvis   ☐ Fatigue

Nutritional Management: *See your nutritionist within 1 month post treatment to develop a plan for optimal nutrition and to manage symptoms* **Contact:** _____

Height: Current Weight: Ideal Body Weight: Weight History:
Weight gain or loss:

Follow up with the Nutritionist to address ongoing concerns related to nutrition, weight status and eating including any of the following symptoms:
☐ Relying on comfort foods   ☐ Changes in taste
☐ Dry/sensitive mouth   ☐ Mouth sores
☐ Changes in taste

Treatment-Related Medications: *Remember to take your medicines as scheduled*

Exams: *Do the appropriate exams as scheduled*
Blood tests: Thyroid function:

Scans:
X-ray: PET/CT: CT: Other:
Self exams:

Integrative Oncology: *Follow up as needed*   **Contact:** _____

☐ Acupuncture
Breath/relaxation techniques: ☐ Guided imagery   ☐ Progressive relaxation   ☐ Autogenics
Energy therapy: ☐ Reiki   ☐ Therapeutic Touch   ☐ Acupressure

Speech and Swallowing: *Practice what you have been taught by our staff*   **Contact:** _____

- Follow up with your speech and swallowing therapist after completing treatment
- If you had surgery, get a baseline swallowing test after your surgeon clears you for eating orally
Speech Evaluation: ☐ Yes ☐ No
Results:
Swallowing Evaluation: ☐ Yes ☐ No
Results:
Acceptable diet choices:
☐ Thin Liquids   ☐ Thick liquids   ☐ Purees
☐ Soft Solids   ☐ Unrestricted diet

Dental Care: *See your dentist for routine checkups*   **Contact:** _____
  ▪ Teeth/gums care: thoroughly brush your teeth; floss carefully and avoid gum irritation
  ▪ Fluoride regimen: apply fluoride if advised
  ▪ Other oral care:

Breathing: *Practice what you have been taught by our staff*
☐

Other:

ADJUSTING TO SURVIVORSHIP

*Contact your social worker if you are experiencing distress
in any of the following areas*   **Contact:** _____

☐ Body-image   ☐ Eating/sleeping patterns   ☐ Disinterest in activities that you enjoy
                                ☐ Relationships with your family
☐ Pervasive concerns and worry   and friends   ☐ Relationship with partner

☐ Changes in mood   ☐ Sadness   ☐ Fears
☐ Nervousness

WELLNESS

Avoid: **Maintain:**
☐ Nicotine and Tobacco Products   ☐ Healthy nutrition
☐ Alcohol use   ☐ Physical activity
☐ Drug use   ☐ Screening for other cancers
☐ Overexposure to the sun

Screening for other cancers:
☐ Colonoscopy   ☐ Mammogram   ☐ PSA/Digital Rectal exam   ☐ PAP/HPV tests   ☐ Skin exam

ADDITIONAL INFORMATION

Organizations/Programs:	Contact Info:	Website:
Alcoholics Anonymous (AA)	Many local groups exist	http://www.alcoholics-anonymous.org
Narcotics Anonymous (NA)	Many local groups exist	http://www.na.org

Cancer Support Groups:	Contact Info:	Website:
American Cancer Society	1-800-ACS-2345	http://www.cancer.org
CancerCare	1-800-813-HOPE	http://www.cancercare.org
People Living With Cancer		http://www.cancer.net
National Cancer Institute (NCI)	1-800-4-CANCER	http://www.cancer.gov
NCI Office of Cancer Survivorship	1-301-402-2964	http://dccps.nci.nih.gov/ocs
Gilda's Club	1-888-GILDA-4-U	http://www.gildasclubnyc.org
LIVESTRONG	1-866-235-7205	http://www.livestrong.org

PERSONAL HEALTH RECORD
SARCOMA

Last Name: First Name:
DOB: Age: Gender: Date:
Day Phone: Evening Phone:
Address: City: State: Zip:
Email:
My Insurance: Policy #:

Spouse/Relative/Caretaker: Phone:
Health Care Agent: Phone:

MEDICAL INFORMATION

Type of cancer: Date of diagnosis:
Staging   T: N: M:

My Health Care Team   Phone: Email:
Medical Oncologist:
Radiation Oncologist:
Thoracic Surgeon:
Fellow:
Pulmonologist:
Nurse/Nurse Practitioner:
Integrative Oncology Nurse:
Pain/Symptom Management:
Social Worker:
Nutritionist:
Physical Therapist:
Patient Navigator:

Treatments received:
Surgical Procedures:

Chemotherapy: ☐ doxorubicin   (mg)   ☐ dacarbazine   (mg)   ☐ mesna   (mg)
☐ gemcitabine   (mg)   ☐ vinorelbine   (mg)   ☐ irinotecan   (mg) ☐ docetaxel   (mg)
                                                                   ☐ other
Freq: Total Dose:
Radiation Therapy:
Area treated:
☐ External Beam Radiation Therapy   Last Date: Dose:
(EBRT)
☐ Brachytherapy   Last Date: Procedure: Dose:

FOLLOW-UP APPOINTMENTS:
Follow-ups: *Remember to follow up with your providers on a regular schedule*

☐ Surgical: ☐ Radiation Oncology: ☐ Medical Oncology:
☐ Cancer Supportive Services:
                               ☐ Pain/Symptom Management: ☐ Nutrition:
☐ Pulmonologist   ☐ Physical Therapy: ☐ Social Work:

IMPORTANT FOLLOW-UP CARE:
Shortness of Breath   Blood when: number per day:
Taper and avoid nicotine products   Avoid alcoholic beverages
Physical Therapy: *Practice the exercises you have been given by our*   Contact: _____
staff to manage the following
☐ Fatigue/general   ☐ Pain   ☐ Shortness of Breath   ☐
deconditioning

Nutritional Management: *See your nutritionist within 1 month post*
treatment to develop a plan for optimal nutrition and to manage symptoms   Contact: _____

Height: Current Weight: Ideal Body Weight: Weight History:
Weight gain or loss:

Follow up with the Nutritionist to address ongoing concerns related to nutrition, weight status and eating including any of the
following symptoms:
☐ Relying on comfort foods   ☐ Breathing exercise; pulmonary rehabilitation
☐ Dry/sensitive mouth   ☐ Mouth sores
☐ Changes in taste

Treatment-Related Medications:	*Remember to take your medicines as scheduled*		

Exams: *Do the appropriate exams as scheduled*
Blood tests: Thyroid function:

Scans:
X-ray: PET/CT: CT: Other:
Self exams:

Integrative Oncology: *Follow up as needed* Contact: _____

☐ Acupuncture
Breath/relaxation techniques: ☐ Guided imagery ☐ Progressive relaxation ☐ Autogenics
Energy therapy: ☐ Reiki ☐ Therapeutic Touch ☐ Acupressure

Speech and Swallowing: *Practice what you have been taught by our staff*
Contact: _____

- Follow up with your speech and swallowing therapist after completing treatment
- If you had surgery, get a baseline swallowing test after your surgeon clears you for eating orally
Speech Evaluation: ☐ Yes ☐ No
Results:
Swallowing Evaluation: ☐ Yes ☐ No
Results:
Acceptable diet choices:
☐ Thin Liquids ☐ Thick liquids ☐ Purees
☐ Soft Solids ☐ Unrestricted diet

Dental Care: *See your dentist for routine checkups* Contact: _____
- Teeth/gums care: thoroughly brush your teeth; floss carefully and avoid gum irritation
- Fluoride regimen: apply fluoride if advised
- Other oral care:

Breathing: *Practice what you have been taught by our staff*
☐

Other:

ADJUSTING TO SURVIVORSHIP

Contact your social worker if you are experiencing distress
in any of the following areas Contact: _____

☐ Body-image ☐ Eating/sleeping patterns ☐ Disinterest in activities that you enjoy
☐ Pervasive concerns and worry ☐ Relationships with your family and friends ☐ Relationship with partner
☐ Changes in mood ☐ Sadness ☐ Fears
☐ Nervousness

WELLNESS

Avoid: Maintain:
☐ Nicotine and Tobacco Products ☐ Healthy nutrition
☐ Alcohol use ☐ Physical activity
☐ Drug use ☐ Screening for other cancers
☐ Overexposure to the sun

Screening for other cancers:
☐ Colonoscopy ☐ Mammogram ☐ PSA/Digital Rectal exam ☐ PAP/HPV tests ☐ Skin exam

ADDITIONAL INFORMATION

Organizations/Programs:	Contact Info:	Website:
Alcoholics Anonymous (AA)	Many local groups exist	http://www.alcoholics-anonymous.org
Narcotics Anonymous (NA)	Many local groups exist	http://www.na.org

Cancer Support Groups:	Contact Info:	Website:
American Cancer Society	1-800-ACS-2345	http://www.cancer.org
CancerCare	1-800-813-HOPE	http://www.cancercare.org
People Living With Cancer		http://www.cancer.net
National Cancer Institute (NCI)	1-800-4-CANCER	http://www.cancer.gov
NCI Office of Cancer Survivorship	1-301-402-2964	http://dccps.nci.nih.gov/ocs
Gilda's Club	1-888-GILDA-4-U	http://www.gildasclubnyc.org
LIVESTRONG	1-866-235-7205	http://www.livestrong.org

PERSONAL HEALTH RECORD
TESTICULAR CANCER

Last Name: First Name:
DOB: Age: Gender: Date:
Day Phone: Evening Phone:
Address: City: State: Zip:
Email:
My Insurance: Policy #:

Spouse/Relative/Caretaker: Phone:
Health Care Agent: Phone:

MEDICAL INFORMATION

Type of cancer: Date of diagnosis:
Staging   T: N: M:

My Health Care Team   **Phone:**   **Email:**
Medical Oncologist:
Radiation Oncologist:
Thoracic Surgeon:
Fellow:
Pulmonologist:
Nurse/Nurse Practitioner:
Integrative Oncology Nurse:
Pain/Symptom Management:
Social Worker:
Nutritionist:
Physical Therapist:
Patient Navigator:
Sperm or testicular banking addressed prior to treatment?

Treatments received:
Surgical Procedures:

Chemotherapy: ☐ etoposide   (mg)   ☐ cisplatin   (mg)   ☐ mesna   (mg)
☐ ifosfamide   (mg)   ☐ bleomycin   (mg) ☐   ☐ other
Freq: Total Dose:

Radiation Therapy:
Area treated:
☐ External Beam Radiation Therapy
(EBRT)   Last Date: Dose:
☐ Brachytherapy   Last Date: Procedure: Dose:

FOLLOW-UP APPOINTMENTS:
Follow-ups: *Remember to follow up with your providers on a regular schedule*

☐ Surgical: ☐ Radiation Oncology: ☐ Medical Oncology:
☐ Cancer Supportive Services:
                             ☐ Pain/Symptom Management: ☐ Nutrition:
☐ Pulmonologist   ☐ Physical Therapy: ☐ Social Work:

IMPORTANT FOLLOW-UP CARE:
Shortness of Breath   Blood whens: number per day
Taper and avoid nicotine products   Avoid alcoholic beverages
Physical Therapy: *Practice the exercises you have been given by our*   **Contact:** _____
staff to manage the following
☐ Fatigue/general   ☐ Pain   ☐ Shortness of Breath   ☐
deconditioning

Nutritional Management: *See your nutritionist within 1 month post*   _____
treatment to develop a plan for optimal nutrition and to manage symptoms   **Contact:**

Height: Current Weight: Ideal Body Weight: Weight History:
Weight gain or loss:

Follow up with the Nutritionist to address ongoing concerns related to nutrition, weight status and eating including any of the
following symptoms:
☐ Relying on comfort foods   ☐ Breathing exercise; pulmonary rehabilitation
☐ Dry/sensitive mouth   ☐ Mouth sores
☐ Changes in taste

Treatment-Related Medications: *Remember to take your medicines as scheduled*

Exams: *Do the appropriate exams as scheduled*
Blood tests: Thyroid function:

Scans:
X-ray: PET/CT: CT: Other:
Self exams:

Integrative Oncology: *Follow up as needed*   **Contact:** _____

☐ Acupuncture
Breath/relaxation techniques: ☐ Guided imagery ☐ Progressive relaxation ☐ Autogenics
Energy therapy: ☐ Reiki   ☐ Therapeutic Touch ☐ Acupressure

Speech and Swallowing: *Practice what you have been taught by our staff* **Contact:** _____

- *Follow up with your speech and swallowing therapist after completing treatment*
- *If you had surgery, get a baseline swallowing test after your surgeon clears you for eating orally*
Speech Evaluation: ☐ Yes ☐ No
Results:
Swallowing Evaluation: ☐ Yes ☐ No
Results:
Acceptable diet choices:
☐ Thin Liquids   ☐ Thick liquids   ☐ Purees
☐ Soft Solids   ☐ Unrestricted diet

Dental Care: *See your dentist for routine checkups* **Contact:** _____
 • Teeth/gums care: thoroughly brush your teeth; floss carefully and avoid gum irritation
 • Fluoride regimen: apply fluoride if advised
 • Other oral care:

Breathing: *Practice what you have been taught by our staff*
☐

Other:

ADJUSTING TO SURVIVORSHIP

*Contact your social worker if you are experiencing distress
in any of the following areas*   **Contact:** _____

☐ Body-image   ☐ Eating/sleeping patterns ☐ Disinterest in activities that you enjoy
☐ Pervasive concerns and worry ☐ Relationships with your family and friends ☐ Relationship with partner
☐ Changes in mood   ☐ Sadness   ☐ Fears
☐ Nervousness

WELLNESS

Avoid: **Maintain:**
☐ Nicotine and Tobacco Products   ☐ Healthy nutrition
☐ Alcohol use   ☐ Physical activity
☐ Drug use   ☐ Screening for other cancers
☐ Overexposure to the sun

Screening for other cancers:
☐ Colonoscopy ☐ Mammogram ☐ PSA/Digital Rectal exam ☐ PAP/HPV tests ☐ Skin exam

ADDITIONAL INFORMATION

Organizations/Programs:	Contact Info:	Website:
Testicular Cancer Awareness Foundation		http://testicularcancerawarenessfoundation.org
Alcoholics Anonymous (AA)	Many local groups exist	http://www.acoholics-anonymous.org
Narcotics Anonymous (NA)	Many local groups exist	http://www.na.org

Cancer Support Groups:	Contact Info:	Website:
American Cancer Society	1-800-ACS-2345	http://www.cancer.org
CancerCare	1-800-813-HOPE	http://www.cancercare.org
People Living With Cancer		http://www.cancer.net
National Cancer Institute (NCI)	1-800-4-CANCER	http://www.cancer.gov
NCI Office of Cancer Survivorship	1-301-402-2964	http://dccps.nci.nih.gov/ocs
Gilda's Club	1-888-GILDA-4-U	http://www.gildasclubnyc.org
LIVESTRONG	1-866-235-7205	http://www.livestrong.org

PERSONAL HEALTH RECORD
THYMOMA

Last Name: First Name:
DOB: Age: Gender: Date:
Day Phone: Evening Phone:
Address: City: State: Zip:
Email:
My Insurance: Policy #:

Spouse/Relative/Caretaker: Phone:
Health Care Agent: Phone:

MEDICAL INFORMATION

Type of cancer: Date of diagnosis:
Staging   Masaoka Stage:

My Health Care Team   **Phone:**   **Email:**
Medical Oncologist:
Radiation Oncologist:
Thoracic Surgeon:
Fellow:
Pulmonologist:
Nurse/Nurse Practitioner:
Integrative Oncology Nurse:
Pain/Symptom Management:
Social Worker:
Nutritionist:
Physical Therapist:
Patient Navigator:

Treatments received:
Surgical Procedures:

Chemotherapy: ☐ doxorubicin   (mg) ☐ cisplatin   (mg) ☐ cyclophosphamide   (mg)
☐ etoposide   (mg)   ☐ ifosfamide   (mg)   ☐ paclitaxel   (mg)
☐ other   Freq: Total Dose:

Radiation Therapy:
Area treated:
☐ External Beam Radiation Therapy   Last Date: Dose:
(EBRT)
☐ Intraopeartive Radiation Therapy   Last Date: Procedure: Dose:

FOLLOW-UP APPOINTMENTS:
Follow-ups: *Remember to follow up with your providers on a regular schedule*

☐ Surgical: ☐ Radiation Oncology: ☐ Medical Oncology:
☐ Cancer Supportive Services: ☐ Pain/Symptom Management: ☐ Nutrition:
☐ Pulmonologist: ☐ Physical Therapy: ☐ Social Work:

IMPORTANT FOLLOW-UP CARE:
Shortness of Breath   Alpha-feto protein (AFP):   beta HCG
Taper and avoid nicotine products   Avoid alcoholic beverages
Physical Therapy: *Practice the exercises you have been given by our*
staff to manage the following   **Contact:** _____
☐ Fatigue/general deconditioning   ☐ Pain   ☐ Shortness of Breath   ☐

Nutritional Management: *See your nutritionist within 1 month post*
treatment to develop a plan for optimal nutrition and to manage symptoms **Contact:** _____

Height: Current Weight: Ideal Body Weight: Weight History:
Weight gain or loss:

Follow up with the Nutritionist to address ongoing concerns related to nutrition, weight status and eating including any of the
following symptoms:
☐ Relying on comfort foods   ☐ Breathing exercise; pulmonary rehabilitation
☐ Dry/sensitive mouth   ☐ Mouth sores
☐ Changes in taste

Treatment-Related Medications: *Remember to take your medicines as scheduled*

Exams: *Do the appropriate exams as scheduled*
Blood tests: Thyroid function:

Scans:
X-ray: PET/CT: CT: Other:
Self exams:

Integrative Oncology: *Follow up as needed* Contact: _____

☐ Acupuncture
Breath/relaxation techniques: ☐ Guided imagery ☐ Progressive relaxation ☐ Autogenics
Energy therapy: ☐ Reiki ☐ Therapeutic Touch ☐ Acupressure

Speech and Swallowing: *Practice what you have been taught by our staff*
Contact: _____

- *Follow up with your speech and swallowing therapist after completing treatment*
- *If you had surgery, get a baseline swallowing test after your surgeon clears you for eating orally*
Speech Evaluation: ☐ Yes ☐ No
Results:
Swallowing Evaluation: ☐ Yes ☐ No
Results:
Acceptable diet choices:
☐ Thin Liquids ☐ Thick liquids ☐ Purees
☐ Soft Solids ☐ Unrestricted diet

Dental Care: *See your dentist for routine checkups* Contact: _____
- Teeth/gums care: thoroughly brush your teeth; floss carefully and avoid gum irritation
- Fluoride regimen: apply fluoride if advised
- Other oral care:

Breathing: *Practice what you have been taught by the staff*
☐

Other:

ADJUSTING TO SURVIVORSHIP

Contact your social worker if you are experiencing distress
in any of the following areas Contact: _____

☐ Body-image ☐ Eating/sleeping patterns ☐ Disinterest in activities that you enjoy
☐ Pervasive concerns and worry ☐ Relationships with your family and friends ☐ Relationship with spouse/partner
☐ Changes in mood ☐ Sadness ☐ Fears
☐ Nervousness

WELLNESS

Avoid: **Maintain:**
☐ Nicotine and Tobacco Products ☐ Healthy nutrition
☐ Alcohol use ☐ Physical activity
☐ Drug use ☐ Screening for other cancers
☐ Overexposure to the sun

Screening for other cancers:
☐ Colonoscopy ☐ Mammogram ☐ PSA/Digital Rectal exam ☐ PAP/HPV tests ☐ Skin exam

ADDITIONAL INFORMATION

Organizations/Programs:	Contact Info:	Website:
Alcoholics Anonymous (AA)	Many local groups exist	http://www.alcoholics-anonymous.org
Narcotics Anonymous (NA)	Many local groups exist	http://www.na.org

Cancer Support Groups:	Contact Info:	Website:
American Cancer Society	1-800-ACS-2345	http://www.cancer.org
CancerCare	1-800-813-HOPE	http://www.cancercare.org
People Living With Cancer		http://www.cancer.net
National Cancer Institute (NCI)	1-800-4-CANCER	http://www.cancer.gov
NCI Office of Cancer Survivorship	1-301-402-2964	http://dccps.nci.nih.gov/ocs
Gilda's Club	1-888-GILDA-4-U	http://www.gildasclubnyc.org
LIVESTRONG	1-866-235-7205	http://www.livestrong.org

MY PERSONAL AFFAIRS

❑ Last will and testament

❑ Health care proxy, living will, or other advance medical directive acceptable in your state

❑ Power of attorney

❑ List of bank accounts, pensions, life insurance policies (with review of the beneficiaries or "in trust for..." designations)

❑ Special accommodations for dependent children or elderly

❑ Thoughts about memorial services, burial or cremation, including list of invitees

❑ Wording of obituary

❑ Letters, audio or video recordings you would like to leave for loved ones on upcoming milestones in their lives: school graduations, marriages, births, or other such momentous personal occasions

❑ "How I want you to remember me" thoughts. Written or recorded. This is something almost always neglected because the people who love you the most are afraid to bring it up to avoid scaring you that you are closer to death than you would believe (another conspiracy of silence thing)

❑ "What I know that you may not": genealogy, family history, stories, Grandma's cookie recipes; whatever is significant in your family's life

❑ "Permission slips": Regarding very personal and deep family issues: permission to move from the family house when the time is right; permission for a spouse to date or remarry (grist for many a made-for-television movie), permission to go back to school to finish a degree. There are many variations on this theme.

❑ Thank you's

Journal Page: My Bucket List

With no distractions or interruptions, think about things that you have always wanted to do but have not yet done and list them here:

FIVE WISHES

There are many things in life that are out of our hands. This Five Wishes document gives you a way to control something very important—how you are treated if you get seriously ill. It is an easy-to-complete form that lets you say exactly what you want. Once it is filled out and properly signed it is valid under the laws of most states.

What Is Five Wishes?

Five Wishes is the first living will that talks about your personal, emotional and spiritual needs as well as your medical wishes. It lets you choose the person you want to make health care decisions for you if you are not able to make them for yourself. Five Wishes lets you say exactly how you wish to be treated if you get seriously ill. It was written with the help of The American Bar Association's Commission on Law and Aging, and the nation's leading experts in end-of-life care. It's also easy to use. All you have to do is check a box, circle a direction, or write a few sentences.

How Five Wishes Can Help You And Your Family

- It lets you talk with your family, friends and doctor about how you want to be treated if you become seriously ill.

- Your family members will not have to guess what you want. It protects them if you become seriously ill, because they won't have to make hard choices without knowing your wishes.

- You can know what your mom, dad, spouse, or friend wants. You can be there for them when they need you most. You will understand what they really want.

How Five Wishes Began

For 12 years, Jim Towey worked closely with Mother Teresa, and, for one year, he lived in a hospice she ran in Washington, DC. Inspired by this first-hand experience, Mr. Towey sought a way for patients and their families to plan ahead and to cope with serious illness. The result is Five Wishes and the response to it has been overwhelming. It has been featured on CNN and NBC's Today Show and in the pages of *Time* and *Money* magazines. Newspapers have called Five Wishes the first "living will with a heart and soul." Today, Five Wishes is available in 23 languages

Who Should Use Five Wishes

Five Wishes is for anyone 18 or older — married, single, parents, adult children, and friends. Over 13 million Americans of all ages have already used it. Because it works so well, lawyers, doctors, hospitals and hospices, faith communities, employer and retiree groups are handing out this document.

Five Wishes States

If you live in the **District of Columbia** or one of the **42 states** listed below, you can use Five Wishes and have the peace of mind to know that it substantially meets your state's requirements under the law:

Alaska	Illinois	Montana	South Carolina
Arizona	Iowa	Nebraska	South Dakota
Arkansas	Kentucky	Nevada	Tennessee
California	Louisiana	New Jersey	Vermont
Colorado	Maine	New Mexico	Virginia
Connecticut	Maryland	New York	Washington
Delaware	Massachusetts	North Carolina	West Virginia
Florida	Michigan	North Dakota	Wisconsin
Georgia	Minnesota	Oklahoma	Wyoming
Hawaii	Mississippi	Pennsylvania	
Idaho	Missouri	Rhode Island	

If your state is not one of the 42 states listed here, Five Wishes does not meet the technical requirements in the statutes of your state. So some doctors in your state may be reluctant to honor Five Wishes. However, many people from states not on this list do complete Five Wishes along with their state's legal form. They find that Five Wishes helps them express all that they want and provides a helpful guide to family members, friends, care givers and doctors. Most doctors and health care professionals know they need to listen to your wishes no matter how you express them.

How Do I Change To Five Wishes?

You may already have a living will or a durable power of attorney for health care. If you want to use Five Wishes instead, all you need to do is fill out and sign a new Five Wishes as directed. As soon as you sign it, it takes away any advance directive you had before. To make sure the right form is used, please do the following:

- Destroy all copies of your old living will or durable power of attorney for health care. Or you can write "revoked" in large letters across the copy you have. Tell your lawyer if he or she helped prepare those old forms for you. *AND*

- Tell your Health Care Agent, family members, and doctor that you have filled out a new Five Wishes. Make sure they know about your new wishes.

WISH 1
The Person I Want To Make Health Care Decisions For Me When I Can't Make Them For Myself.

*I*f I am no longer able to make my own health care decisions, this form names the person I choose to make these choices for me. This person will be my Health Care Agent (or other term that may be used in my state, such as proxy, representative, or surrogate). This person will make my health care choices if both of these things happen:

- *My attending or treating doctor finds I am no longer able to make health care choices, AND*
- *Another health care professional agrees that this is true.*

If my state has a different way of finding that I am not able to make health care choices, then my state's way should be followed.

The Person I Choose As My Health Care Agent Is:

First Choice Name

Phone

Address

City/State/Zip

If this person is not able or willing to make these choices for me, *OR* is divorced or legally separated from me, *OR* this person has died, then these people are my next choices:

Second Choice Name

Third Choice Name

Address

Address

City/State/Zip

City/State/Zip

Phone

Phone

Picking The Right Person To Be Your Health Care Agent

Choose someone who knows you very well, cares about you, and who can make difficult decisions. A spouse or family member may not be the best choice because they are too emotionally involved. Sometimes they **are** the best choice. You know best. Choose someone who is able to stand up for you so that your wishes are followed. Also, choose someone who is likely to be nearby so that they can help when you need them. Whether you choose a spouse, family member, or friend as your Health Care Agent, make sure you talk about these wishes and be sure that this person agrees to respect

and follow your wishes. Your Health Care Agent should be **at least 18 years or older** (in Colorado, 21 years or older) and should **not** be:

- Your health care provider, including the owner or operator of a health or residential or community care facility serving you.

- An employee or spouse of an employee of your health care provider.

- Serving as an agent or proxy for 10 or more people unless he or she is your spouse or close relative.

I understand that my Health Care Agent can make health care decisions for me. I want my Agent to be able to do the following: (**Please cross out anything you don't want your Agent to do that is listed below.**)

- Make choices for me about my medical care or services, like tests, medicine, or surgery. This care or service could be to find out what my health problem is, or how to treat it. It can also include care to keep me alive. If the treatment or care has already started, my Health Care Agent can keep it going or have it stopped.

- Interpret any instructions I have given in this form or given in other discussions, according to my Health Care Agent's understanding of my wishes and values.

- Consent to admission to an assisted living facility, hospital, hospice, or nursing home for me. My Health Care Agent can hire any kind of health care worker I may need to help me or take care of me. My Agent may also fire a health care worker, if needed.

- Make the decision to request, take away or not give medical treatments, including artificially-provided food and water, and any other treatments to keep me alive.

- See and approve release of my medical records and personal files. If I need to sign my name to get any of these files, my Health Care Agent can sign it for me.

- Move me to another state to get the care I need or to carry out my wishes.

- Authorize or refuse to authorize any medication or procedure needed to help with pain.

- Take any legal action needed to carry out my wishes.

- Donate useable organs or tissues of mine as allowed by law.

- Apply for Medicare, Medicaid, or other programs or insurance benefits for me. My Health Care Agent can see my personal files, like bank records, to find out what is needed to fill out these forms.

- Listed below are any changes, additions, or limitations on my Health Care Agent's powers.

_____
_____
_____
_____
_____
_____

If I Change My Mind About Having A Health Care Agent, I Will

- Destroy all copies of this part of the Five Wishes form. *OR*

- Tell someone, such as my doctor or family, that I want to cancel or change my Health Care Agent. *OR*

- Write the word "Revoked" in large letters across the name of each agent whose authority I want to cancel. Sign my name on that page.

WISH 2
My Wish For The Kind Of Medical Treatment
I Want Or Don't Want.

I believe that my life is precious and I deserve to be treated with dignity. When the time comes that I am very sick and am not able to speak for myself, I want the following wishes, and any other directions I have given to my Health Care Agent, to be respected and followed.

What You Should Keep In Mind As My Caregiver

- I do not want to be in pain. I want my doctor to give me enough medicine to relieve my pain, even if that means that I will be drowsy or sleep more than I would otherwise.

- I do not want **anything done or omitted by my doctors or nurses with the intention of taking my life.**

- **I want to be offered food and fluids by mouth, and kept clean and warm.**

What "Life-Support Treatment" Means To Me

Life-support treatment means any medical procedure, device or medication to keep me alive. Life-support treatment includes: medical devices put in me to help me breathe; food and water supplied by medical device (tube feeding); cardiopulmonary resuscitation (CPR); major surgery; blood transfusions; dialysis; antibiotics; and anything else meant to keep me alive. If I wish to limit the meaning of life-support treatment because of my religious or personal beliefs, I write this limitation in the space below. I do this to make very clear what I want and under what conditions.

_____

_____

_____

_____

_____

In Case Of An Emergency

If you have a medical emergency and ambulance personnel arrive, they may look to see if you have a **Do Not Resuscitate** form or bracelet. Many states require a person to have a **Do Not Resuscitate** form filled out and signed by a doctor. This form lets ambulance personnel know that you don't want them to use life-support treatment when you are dying. Please check with your doctor to see if you need to have a **Do Not Resuscitate** form filled out.

Here is the kind of medical treatment that I want or don't want in the four situations listed below. I want my Health Care Agent, my family, my doctors and other health care providers, my friends and all others to know these directions.

Close to death:

If my doctor and another health care professional both decide that I am likely to die within a short period of time, and life-support treatment would only delay the moment of my death (Choose *one* of the following):

☐ I want to have life-support treatment.

☐ I do not want life-support treatment. If it has been started, I want it stopped.

☐ I want to have life-support treatment if my doctor believes it could help. But I want my doctor to stop giving me life-support treatment if it is not helping my health condition or symptoms.

In A Coma And Not Expected To Wake Up Or Recover:

If my doctor and another health care professional both decide that I am in a coma from which I am not expected to wake up or recover, and I have brain damage, and life-support treatment would only delay the moment of my death (Choose *one* of the following):

☐ I want to have life-support treatment.

☐ I do not want life-support treatment. If it has been started, I want it stopped.

☐ I want to have life-support treatment if my doctor believes it could help. But I want my doctor to stop giving me life-support treatment if it is not helping my health condition or symptoms.

Permanent And Severe Brain Damage And Not Expected To Recover:

If my doctor and another health care professional both decide that I have permanent and severe brain damage, (for example, I can open my eyes, but I can not speak or understand) and I am not expected to get better, and life-support treatment would only delay the moment of my death (Choose *one* of the following):

☐ I want to have life-support treatment.

☐ I do not want life-support treatment. If it has been started, I want it stopped.

☐ I want to have life-support treatment if my doctor believes it could help. But I want my doctor to stop giving me life-support treatment if it is not helping my health condition or symptoms.

In Another Condition Under Which I Do Not Wish To Be Kept Alive:

If there is another condition under which I do not wish to have life-support treatment, I describe it below. In this condition, I believe that the costs and burdens of life-support treatment are too much and not worth the benefits to me. Therefore, in this condition, I do not want life-support treatment. (For example, you may write "end-stage condition." That means that your health has gotten worse. You are not able to take care of yourself in any way, mentally or physically. Life-support treatment will not help you recover. Please leave the space blank if you have no other condition to describe.)

_____
_____
_____
_____
_____

*T*he next three wishes deal with my personal, spiritual and emotional wishes. They are important to me. I want to be treated with dignity near the end of my life, so I would like people to do the things written in Wishes 3, 4, and 5 when they can be done. I understand that my family, my doctors and other health care providers, my friends, and others may not be able to do these things or are not required by law to do these things. I do not expect the following wishes to place new or added legal duties on my doctors or other health care providers. I also do not expect these wishes to excuse my doctor or other health care providers from giving me the proper care asked for by law.

WISH 3
My Wish For How Comfortable I Want To Be.
(Please cross out anything that you don't agree with.)

- I do not want to be in pain. I want my doctor to give me enough medicine to relieve my pain, even if that means I will be drowsy or sleep more than I would otherwise.

- If I show signs of depression, nausea, shortness of breath, or hallucinations, I want my care givers to do whatever they can to help me.

- I wish to have a cool moist cloth put on my head if I have a fever.

- I want my lips and mouth kept moist to stop dryness.

- I wish to have warm baths often. I wish to be kept fresh and clean at all times.

- I wish to be massaged with warm oils as often as I can be.

- I wish to have my favorite music played when possible until my time of death.

- I wish to have personal care like shaving, nail clipping, hair brushing, and teeth brushing, as long as they do not cause me pain or discomfort.

- I wish to have religious readings and well-loved poems read aloud when I am near death.

- I wish to know about options for hospice care to provide medical, emotional and spiritual care for me and my loved ones.

WISH 4
My Wish For How I Want People To Treat Me.
(Please cross out anything that you don't agree with.)

- I wish to have people with me when possible. I want someone to be with me when it seems that death may come at any time.

- I wish to have my hand held and to be talked to when possible, even if I don't seem to respond to the voice or touch of others.

- I wish to have others by my side praying for me when possible.

- I wish to have the members of my faith community told that I am sick and asked to pray for me and visit me.

- I wish to be cared for with kindness and cheerfulness, and not sadness.

- I wish to have pictures of my loved ones in my room, near my bed.

- If I am not able to control my bowel or bladder functions, I wish for my clothes and bed linens to be kept clean, and for them to be changed as soon as they can be if they have been soiled.

- I want to die in my home, if that can be done.

WISH 5

My Wish For What I Want My Loved Ones To Know.

(Please cross out anything that you don't agree with.)

- I wish to have my family and friends know that I love them.

- I wish to be forgiven for the times I have hurt my family, friends, and others.

- I wish to have my family, friends and others know that I forgive them for when they may have hurt me in my life.

- I wish for my family and friends to know that I do not fear death itself. I think it is not the end, but a new beginning for me.

- I wish for all of my family members to make peace with each other before my death, if they can.

- I wish for my family and friends to think about what I was like before I became seriously ill. I want them to remember me in this way after my death.

- I wish for my family and friends and caregivers to respect my wishes even if they don't agree with them.

- I wish for my family and friends to look at my dying as a time of personal growth for everyone, including me. This will help me live a meaningful life in my final days.

- I wish for my family and friends to get counseling if they have trouble with my death. I want memories of my life to give them joy and not sorrow.

- After my death, I would like my body to be (circle one): buried   or   cremated.

- My body or remains should be put in the following location_____.

- The following person knows my funeral wishes: _____.

If anyone asks how I want to be remembered, please say the following about me:

_____

_____

_____

If there is to be a memorial service for me, I wish for this service to include the following (list music, songs, readings or other specific requests that you have):

_____

_____

_____

(Please use the space below for any other wishes. For example, you may want to donate any or all parts of your body when you die. You may also wish to designate a charity to receive memorial contributions. Please attach a separate sheet of paper if you need more space.)

_____

_____

_____

Signing The Five Wishes Form

Please make sure you sign your Five Wishes form in the presence of the two witnesses.

I, _____, ask that my family, my doctors, and other health care providers, my friends, and all others, follow my wishes as communicated by my Health Care Agent (if I have one and he or she is available), or as otherwise expressed in this form. This form becomes valid when I am unable to make decisions or speak for myself. If any part of this form cannot be legally followed, I ask that all other parts of this form be followed. I also revoke any health care advance directives I have made before.

Signature: _____

Address: _____

Phone: _____ Date: _____

Witness Statement • (2 witnesses needed):

I, the witness, declare that the person who signed or acknowledged this form (hereafter "person") is personally known to me, that he/she signed or acknowledged this [Health Care Agent and/or Living Will form(s)] in my presence, and that he/she appears to be of sound mind and under no duress, fraud, or undue influence.

I also declare that I am over 18 years of age and am NOT:

- The individual appointed as (agent/proxy/surrogate/patient advocate/representative) by this document or his/her successor,
- The person's health care provider, including owner or operator of a health, long-term care, or other residential or community care facility serving the person,
- An employee of the person's health care provider,

- Financially responsible for the person's health care,
- An employee of a life or health insurance provider for the person,
- Related to the person by blood, marriage, or adoption, and,
- To the best of my knowledge, a creditor of the person or entitled to any part of his/her estate under a will or codicil, by operation of law.

(Some states may have fewer rules about who may be a witness. Unless you know your state's rules, please follow the above.)

Signature of Witness #1	Signature of Witness #2
Printed Name of Witness	Printed Name of Witness
Address	Address
Phone	Phone

Notarization • Only required for residents of Missouri, North Carolina, South Carolina and West Virginia

- If you live in Missouri, only your signature should be notarized.

- If you live in North Carolina, South Carolina or West Virginia, you should have your signature, and the signatures of your witnesses, notarized.

STATE OF_____   COUNTY OF_____

On this _____ day of _____, 20_____, the said _____,
_____, and _____, known to me (or satisfactorily proven) to be the person named in the
,oing instrument and witnesses, respectively, personally appeared before me, a Notary Public, within and for the State and County aforesaid, and
acknowledged that they freely and voluntarily executed the same for the purposes stated therein.

My Commission Expires: _____

10   Notary Public

What To Do After You Complete Five Wishes

- Make sure you sign and witness the form just the way it says in the directions. Then your Five Wishes will be legal and valid.

- Talk about your wishes with your health care agent, family members and others who care about you. Give them copies of your completed Five Wishes.

- Keep the original copy you signed in a special place in your home. Do NOT put it in a safe deposit box. Keep it nearby so that someone can find it when you need it.

- Fill out the wallet card below. Carry it with you. That way people will know where you keep your Five Wishes.

- Talk to your doctor during your next office visit. Give your doctor a copy of your Five Wishes. Make sure it is put in your medical record. Be sure your doctor understands your wishes and is willing to follow them. Ask him or her to tell other doctors who treat you to honor them.

- If you are admitted to a hospital or nursing home, take a copy of your Five Wishes with you. Ask that it be put in your medical record.

- I have given the following people copies of my completed Five Wishes:

  _____

  _____

  _____

Residents of WISCONSIN must attach the WISCONSIN notice statement to Five Wishes.
More information and the notice statement are available at www.agingwithdignity.org or 1-888-594-7437.

Residents of Institutions In CALIFORNIA, CONNECTICUT, DELAWARE, GEORGIA, NEW YORK, NORTH DAKOTA, SOUTH CAROLINA, and VERMONT Must Follow Special Witnessing Rules.

If you live in certain institutions (a nursing home, other licensed long term care facility, a home for the mentally retarded or developmentally disabled, or a mental health institution) in one of the states listed above, you may have to follow special "witnessing requirements" for your Five Wishes to be valid. For further information, please contact a social worker or patient advocate at your institution.

Five Wishes is meant to help you plan for the future. It is not meant to give you legal advice. It does not try to answer all questions about anything that could come up. Every person is different, and every situation is different. Laws change from time to time. If you have a specific question or problem, talk to a medical or legal professional for advice.

Five Wishes Wallet Card

✂ -

Important Notice to Medical Personnel:
I have a Five Wishes Advance Directive.

Signature
_____

Please consult this document and/or my Health Care Agent in an emergency. My Agent is:

Name
_____

Address   City/State/Zip

Phone

My primary care physician is:

Name
_____

Address   City/State/Zip

Phone

My document is located at:

_____

_____

_____

Cut Out Card, Fold and Laminate for Safekeeping

Here's What People Are Saying About Five Wishes:

"It will be a year since my mother passed on. We knew what she wanted because she had the Five Wishes living will. When it came down to the end, my brother and I had no questions on what we needed to do. We had peace of mind."

Cheryl K.
Longwood, Florida

"I must say I love your Five Wishes. It's clear, easy to understand, and doesn't dwell on the concrete issues of medical care, but on the issues of real importance—human care. I used it for myself and my husband."

Susan W.
Flagstaff, Arizona

"I don't want my children to have to make the decisions I am having to make for my mother. I never knew that there were so many medical options to be considered. Thank you for such a sensitive and caring form. I can simply fill it out and have it on file for my children."

Diana W.
Hanover, Illinois

To Order:

Call (888) 5-WISHES to purchase more copies of Five Wishes, the Five Wishes DVD, or Next Steps guides. Ask about the "Family Package" that includes 10 Five Wishes, 2 Next Steps guides and 1 DVD at a savings of more than 50%. For more information visit Aging with Dignity's website, or call for details.

(888) 5-WISHES or (888) 594-7437
www.agingwithdignity.org

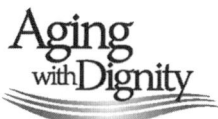

P.O. Box 1661
Tallahassee, Florida 32302-1661

References

1a. Institute of Medicine. *From Cancer Patient to Cancer Survivor: Lost in Transition.* Washington, DC: The National Academies Press; 2006.

1b. Mariotto AB, Yabroff KR, Shao Y, Feuer EJ, Brown ML. Projections of the cost of cancer care in the United States: 2010–2020. *J Natl Cancer Inst.* 2011; 103(2):117–128.

2. Clark EJ, Stovall EL, Leigh S, Siu AL, Austin DK, Rowland JH. *Imperatives for Quality Cancer Care: Access, Advocacy, Action, and Accountability.* Silver Spring, MD: National Coalition for Cancer Survivorship; 1996.

3. Mullan F. Seasons of survival: reflections of a physician with cancer. *N Engl J Med.* 1985;313(4):270–273.

4. Poonacha TK, Go RS. Level of scientific evidence underlying recommendations arising from the National Comprehensive Cancer Network clinical practice guidelines. *J Clin Oncol.* 2011;29(2):186–191.

5. Holtzman J, Schmitz K, Babes G, et al. *Effectiveness of Behavioral Interventions to Modify Physical Activity Behaviors in General Populations and Cancer Patients and Survivors.* Rockville, MD: Agency for Healthcare Research and Quality; 2004. Evidence Reports/Technology Assessments, No. 102.

6. Temel JS, Greer JA, Muzikansky A, et al. Early palliative care for patients with metastatic non–small-cell lung cancer. *N Eng J Med.* 2010;363(8):733–742.

7. Bruera E, Hui D. Integrating supportive and palliative care in the trajectory of cancer: establishing goals and models of care. *J Clin Oncol.* 2010;28(25):4013–4017.

8. Stubblefield MD, O'Dell MW, eds. *Cancer Rehabilitation: Principles and Practice.* New York, NY: Demos Medical Publishing; 2009.

9. Holland JC, Rowland JH. *Handbook of Psychooncology: Psychological Care of the Patient with Cancer.* New York, NY: Oxford University Press; 1989.

10. Aktas A, Walsh D, Rybicki L. Symptom clusters: myth or reality? *Palliat Med.* 2010;24(4):373–385.

11. Cheung WY, Le LW, Zimmermann C. Symptom clusters in patients with advanced cancers [published online ahead of print January 30, 2009]. *Support Care Cancer.* 2009;17(9):1223–1230.

12. Kramer BS. The National Institutes of Health State-of-the-Science. Conference on symptom management in cancer: pain, depression and fatigue. *J Natl Cancer Inst.* 2004;32:1–158.

13. Lichtenstein AH, Appel LJ, Brands M, et al. Diet and lifestyle recommendations revision 2006: a scientific statement from the American Heart Association Nutrition Committee. *Circulation.* 2006;114(1):82–96.

14. U.S. Department of Agriculture, U.S. Department of Health and Human Services. *Dietary Guidelines for Americans, 2010.* 7th ed. Washington, DC: U.S. Government Printing Office; 2010.

15. Buckman R. *How to Break Bad News: A Guide for Health Care Professionals.* Baltimore, MD: The Johns Hopkins University Press; 1992.

16. Baile WF, Beale EA. Giving bad news to cancer patients: matching process and content. *J Clin Oncol.* 2003;21(9 suppl):49s–51s.

17. National Comprehensive Cancer Network. Adult cancer pain guidelines. http://www.nccn.org/professionals/physician_gls/pdf/pain.pdf. Accessed April 4, 2011.

18. Dy SM, Lorenz KA, Naeim A, Sanati H, Walling A, Asch SM. Evidence-based recommendations for cancer fatigue, anorexia, depression, and dyspnea. *J Clin Oncol.* 2008;26(23):3886–3895.

19. Fleishman SB, Dressler C, Herndon JE, et al. Quality of life (QOL) advantage of sclerosis for malignant pleural effusion (MPE) via talc thoracoscopy over chest tube infusion of talc slurry: cancer and leukemia Group B study 9334. *Proc ASCO.* 2002;21:1418.

20. Alba AS, Kim H, Whiteson JH, Bartels MN. Cardiopulmonary rehabilitation and cancer rehabilitation. 2. Pulmonary rehabilitation review. *Arch Phys Med Rehabil.* 2006;87(3 suppl 1):S57–S64.

21. Rizos Ch, Papassava M, Golias Ch, Charalabopoulos K. Alcohol consumption and prostate cancer: a mini review. *Exp Oncol.* 2010;32(2):66–70.

22. American Society of Clinical Oncology. Building and maintaining a referral base. *J Oncol Pract.* 2007;3(4):227–230.

23. American Society of Clinical Oncology. Chemotherapy treatment plan and summary. http://www.asco.org/ASCOv2/Practice+%26+Guidelines/Quality+Care/Quality+Measurement+%26+Improvement/Chemotherapy+Treatment+Plan+and+Summary. Accessed March 16, 2011.

24. Journey Forward Web site. http://journeyforward.org. Accessed March 16, 2011.

25. Hahn EE, Ganz PA. Survivorship programs and care plans in practice: variations on a theme. *J Oncol Pract.* 2011;7(2):70–75. doi:10.1200/JOP.2010.000115

26. Nekhlyudov L. "Doc, should I see you or my oncologist?": a primary care perspective on opportunities and challenges in providing comprehensive care for cancer survivors. *J Clin Oncol.* 2009;27(15):2424–2426.

27. Shulman LN, Jacobs LA, Greenfield S, et al. Cancer care and cancer survivorship care in the United States: will we be able to care for these patients in the future? *J Oncol Pract.* 2009;5(3):119–123.

28. American Heart Association. Identifying stages of changes for smoking cessation counseling. http://www.americanheart.org/downloadable/heart/1137710068117StagesOfChange.pdf. Accessed March 19, 2011.

29. Coaching for development certificate course. The Center for Creative Leadership; August, 2007; Greensboro, NC.

30. Altilio T, Fleishman SB, Otis-Green S. Language, the literature, and the patient. *Oncology (Williston Park).* 2005;19(11):1420.

31. Ditto PH, Smucker WD, Danks JH, et al. Stability of older adults' preferences for life-sustaining medical treatment. *Health Psychol.* 2003;22(6):605–615.

32. Chau NG, Zimmerman C, Ma C, Taback N, Krzyzanowska MK. Bereavement practices of physicians in oncology and palliative care. *Arch Intern Med.* 2009;169(10):963–971.

33. National Comprehensive Cancer Network. NCCN clinical practice guidelines in oncology: distress management V.1.2010. http://www.nccn.org. Accessed April 8, 2011.

34. Ludwig DS, Kabat-Zinn J. Mindfulness in medicine. *JAMA*. 2008;300(11): 1350–1352.

35. Korones DN. Living in the moment. *J Clin Oncol*. 2010;28(31):4778–4779.

36. Burton LA, Handzo GF, eds. *Health Care Chaplaincy in Oncology*. New York, NY: Taylor & Francis; 1993.

37. Oncology Nursing Society. Clinical practice resources. http://www.ons.org/ClinicalResources. Accessed March 7, 2011.

38. Karvinen KH, DuBose KD, Carney B, Allison RR. Promotion of physical activity among oncologists in the United States. *J Support Oncol*. 2010;8(1):35–41.

39. Schmitz KH, Courneya KS, Matthews C, et al. American College of Sports Medicine roundtable on exercise guidelines for cancer survivors. *Med Sci Sports Exerc*. 2010;42(7):1409–1426.

40. Pekmezi DW, Demark-Wahnefried W. Updated evidence in support of diet and exercise interventions in cancer survivors [published online ahead of print November 24, 2010]. *Acta Oncol*. 2011;50(2):167–178.

41. Clarkson PM, Kaufman SA. Should resistance exercise be recommended during breast cancer treatment? *Med Hypotheses*. 2010;75(2):192–195.

42. Jones LW, Peppercorn J, Scott JM, Battaglini C. Exercise therapy in the management of solid tumors. *Curr Treat Options Oncol*. 2010;11(1–2):45–58.

43. Speck RM, Courneya KS, Mâsse LC, Duval S, Schmitz KH. An update of controlled physical activity trials in cancer survivors: a systematic review and meta-analysis. *J Cancer Surviv*. 2010;4(2):87–100.

44. Knols R, Aaronson NK, Daniel Uebelhart D. Physical Exercise in Cancer Patients During and After Medical Treatment: A Systematic Review of Randomized and Controlled Clinical Trials. *J Clin Oncol*. 2005;25(16):3830–3842.

45. Cruciani RA, Dvorkin E, Homel P, et al. L-carnitine supplementation in cancer patients with fatigue and carnitine deficiency. Paper presented at: 2004 ASCO Annual Meeting; June 5–8, 2004; New Orleans, LA.

46. Davis MP, Walsh D. Mechanisms of fatigue. *J Support Oncol*. 2010;8(4): 164–174.

47. Inagaki M, Isono M, Okuyama T, et al. Plasma interleukin-6 and fatigue in terminally ill cancer patients. *J Pain Symptom Manage*. 2008;35(2):153–161.

48. Harrington CB, Hansen JA, Moskowitz M, et al. It's not over when it's over: long-term symptoms in cancer survivors—a systematic review. *Int J Psychiatry Med*. 2010;40(2):163–181.

49. Rogers LQ, Hopkins-Price P, Vicari S, et al. Physical activity and health outcomes three months after completing a physical activity behavior change intervention: persistent and delayed effects. *Cancer Epidemiol Biomarkers Prev*. 2009;18(5):1410–1418.

50. Taskila T, de Boer AG, van Dijk FJ, Verbeek JH. Fatigue and its correlates in cancer patients who had returned to work—a cohort study [published online ahead of print September 5, 2010]. *Psychooncology*. 2010.

51. National Comprehensive Cancer Network. NCCN clinical practice guidelines in oncology: cancer-related fatigue V.1.2011. http://www.pfizerpro.com/resources/minisites/oncology/docs/NCCNFatigueGuidelines.pdf

52. Cahill BA. Management of cancer pain. In: Yarbro CH, Frogge MH, Goodman M, eds. *Cancer Nursing Principles and Practice*. 6th ed. Sudbury, MA: Jones & Bartlett Publishers; 2005:662–697.

53. Dalal S, Melzack R. Potentiation of opioid analgesia by psychostimulant drugs: a review. *J Pain Symptom Manage*. 1998;16(4):245–253.

54. Wagner LI, Cella D. Fatigue in cancer: causes, prevalence and treatment approaches. *Br J Cancer*. 2004;91(5):822–828.

55. Lasheen W, Walsh D, Mahmoud F, Davis MP, Rivera N, Khoshknabi DS. Methylphenidate side effects in advanced cancer: a retrospecive analysis. *Am J Hosp Palliat Care*. 2010;27(1):16–23.

56. Lower EE, Fleishman S, Cooper A, et al. Efficacy of dexmethylphenidate for the treatment of fatigue after cancer chemotherapy: a randomized clinical trial. *J Pain Symptom Manage*. 2009;38(5):650–662.

57. Cooper MR, Bird HM, Steinberg M. Efficacy and safety of modafinil in the treatment of cancer-related fatigue. *Ann Pharmacother*. 2009;43(4):721–725.

58. Palesh OG, Roscoe JA, Mustian KM, et al. Prevalence, demographics, and psychological associations of sleep disruption in patients with cancer: University of Rochester Cancer Center–Community Clinical Oncology Program. *J Clin Oncol*. 2010;28(2):292–298.

59. Barichello E, Sawada NO, Sonobe HM, Zago MM. Quality of sleep in postoperative surgical oncology patients. *Rev Lat Am Enfermagem*. 2009;17(4):481–488.

60. Sprod LK, Palesh OG, Janelsins MC, et al. Exercise, sleep quality, and mediators of sleep in breast and prostate cancer patients receiving radiation therapy. *Community Oncol*. 2010;7(10):463–471.

61. Gibbins J, McCoubrie R, Kendrick AH, Senior-Smith G, Davies AN, Hanks GW. Sleep-wake disturbances in patients with advanced cancer and their family carers. *J Pain Symptom Manage*. 2009;38(6):860–870.

62. Berger AM, Kuhn BR, Farr LA, et al. One-year outcomes of a behavioral therapy intervention trial on sleep quality and cancer-related fatigue. *J Clin Oncol*. 2009;27(35):6033–6040.

63. Reed, VA. Shift work, light at night, and the risk of breast cancer. *AAOHN J*. 2011;59(1):37–45.

64. Cutando A, Aneiros-Fernández J, Aneiros-Cachaza J, Arias-Santaigo S. Melatonin and cancer: current knowledge and its approach to oral cavity tumours [published online ahead of print February 2, 2011]. *J Oral Pathol Med*. 2011;40(8):593–597.

65. Desmarais JE, Looper KJ. Interactions between tamoxifen and antidepressants via cytochrome P450 2D6. *J Clin Psychiatry*. 2009;70(12):1688–1697.

66. American Cancer Society. Complementary and alternative methods for cancer management. http://www.cancer.org/Treatment/TreatmentsandSideEffects/ComplementaryandAlternativeMedicine/complementary-and-alternative-methods-for-cancer-management. Accessed March 5, 2011.

67. Dewys WD, Begg C, Lavin PT, et al. Prognostic effect of weight loss prior to chemotherapy in cancer patients. Eastern Cooperative Oncology Group. *Am J Med.* 1980;69(4):491–497.

68. Bennani-Baiti N, Walsh D. What is the cancer anorexia-cachexia syndrome? A historical perspective. *J R Coll Physicians Edinb.* 2009;39(3):257–262.

69. Lasheen W, Walsh D. The cancer anorexia-cachexia syndrome: myth or reality? *Support Care Cancer.* 2010;18(2):265–272.

70. Tisdale MJ. Cancer cachexia. *Curr Opin Gastroenterol.* 2010;26(2):146–151.

71. Lazenby JM, Saif MW. Palliative care from the beginning of treatment for advanced pancreatic cancer. Paper presented at: 2010 ASCO Gastrointestinal Cancers Symposium; January 22–24, 2010; Orlando, FL.

72. Gioulbasanis I, Baracos VE, Giannousi Z, et al. Baseline nutritional evaluation in metastatic lung cancer patients: mini nutritional assessment versus weight loss history [published online ahead of print October 11, 2010]. *Ann Oncol.* 2011;22(4):835–841.

73. Gabison R, Gibbs M, Uziely B, Ganz FD. The cachexia assessment scale: development and psychometric properties. *Oncol Nurs Forum.* 2010;37(5):635–640.

74. Grotenhuis BA, Wijnhoven BP, Hötte GJ, van der Stok EP, Tilanus HW, van Lanschot JJ. Prognostic value of body mass index on short-term and long-term outcome after resection of esophageal cancer. *World J Surg.* 2010;34(11):2621–2627.

75. Lai CC, You JF, Yeh CY, et al. Low preoperative serum albumin in colon cancer: a risk factor for poor outcome. *Int J Colorectal Dis.* 2011;26(4):473–481. doi:10.1007/s00384-010-1113-4

76. Prado CM, Birdsell LA, Baracos VE. The emerging role of computerized tomography in assessing cancer cachexia. *Curr Opin Support Palliat Care.* 2009; 3(4):269–275.

77. Roxburgh CS, McMillan DC. Role of systemic inflammatory response in predicting survival in patients with primary operable cancer. *Future Oncol.* 2010;6(1):149–163.

78. Gharote HP, Mody RN. Estimation of serum leptin in oral squamous cell carcinoma. *J Oral Pathol Med.* 2010;39(1):69–73.

79. Strasser F, Lutz TA, Maeder MT, et al. Safety, tolerability and pharmacokinetics of intravenous ghrelin for cancer-related anorexia/cachexia: a randomised, placebo-controlled, double-blind, double-crossover study. *Br J Cancer.* 2008;98(2):300–308.

80. Grossberg AJ, Scarlett JM, Marks DL. Hypothalamic mechanisms in cachexia [published online ahead of print March 25, 2010]. *Physiol Behav.* 2010; 100(5):478–489.

81. Dodson S, Baracos VE, Jatoi A, et al. Muscle wasting in cancer cachexia: clinical implications, diagnosis, and emerging treatment strategies. *Annu Rev Med.* 2011;62:265–279.

82. American Cancer Society. Chemotherapy principles: an in-depth discussion. http://www.cancer.org/Treatment/TreatmentsandSideEffects/TreatmentTypes/ Chemotherapy/ChemotherapyPrinciplesAnIn-depthDiscussionoftheTechniques anditsRoleinTreatment/chemotherapy-principles-selecting-chemo-drugs-to-use.

83. Ströhle A, Zänker K, Hahn A. Nutrition in oncology: the case of micronutrients (review). *Oncol Rep.* 2010;24(4):815–828.

84. Hutton JL, Martin L, Field CJ, et al. Dietary patterns in patients with advanced cancer: implications for anorexia-cachexia therapy. *Am J Clin Nutr.* 2006;84(5):1163–1170.

85. Bruera E, Strasser F, Palmer JL, et al. Effect of fish oil on appetite and other symptoms in patients with advanced cancer and anorexia/cachexia: a double-blind, placebo-controlled study. *J Clin Oncol.* 2003;21(1):129–134.

86. Wigmore SJ, Barber MD, Ross JA, Tisdale MJ, Fearon KC. Effect of oral eicosapentaenoic acid on weight loss in patients with pancreatic cancer. *Nutr Cancer.* 2000;36(2):177–184.

87. Weed HG, Ferguson ML, Gaff RL, Hustead DS, Nelson JL, Voss AC. Lean body mass gain in patients with head and neck squamous cell cancer treated perioperatively with a protein- and energy-dense nutritional supplement containing eicosapentaenoic acid [published online ahead of print October 21, 2010]. *Head Neck.* 2011;33(7):1027–2033.

88. Macdonald N. Cancer cachexia and targeting chronic inflammation: a unified approach to cancer treatment and palliative/supportive care. *J Support Oncol.* 2007;5(4):157–162.

89. Jatoi A, Rowland K, Loprinzi CL, et al. An eicosapentaenoic acid supplement versus megestrol acetate versus both for patients with cancer-associated wasting: a North Central Cancer Treatment Group and National Cancer Institute of Canada collaborative effort. *J Clin Oncol.* 2004;22(12):2469–2476.

90. Lundholm K, Körner U, Gunnebo L, et al. Insulin treatment in cancer cachexia: effects on survival, metabolism, and physical functioning. *Clin Cancer Res.* 2007;13(9):2699–2706.

91. Nissen SL, Abumrad NN. Nutritional role of leucine metabolite β-hydroxy β-methylbutyrate (HMB). *J Nutr Biochem.* 1997;8(6):300–311.

92. May PE, Barber A, D'Olimpio JT, Hourihane A, Abumrad NN. Reversal of cancer-related wasting using oral supplementation with a combination of beta-hyroxy-beta-methylbutyrate, arginine, and glutamine. *Am J Surg.* 2002;183(4):471–479.

93. Kosty MP, Fleishman SB, Herndon JE II, et al. Cisplatin, vinblastine, and hydrazine sulfate in advanced non–small-cell lung cancer: a randomized placebo-controlled, double-blind phase III study of the cancer and leukemia group B. *J Clin Oncol.* 1994;12(6):1113–1120.

94. Fleishman SB, Chadha JS. Weight and appetite loss in cancer. In: Holland JC, Breitbart WS, Jacobsen PB, Lederberg MS, Loscalzo MJ, Mccorkle RS, eds. *Psycho-Oncology.* 2nd ed. New York, NY: Oxford University Press; 2010:270–277.

95. Granda-Cameron C, DeMille D, Lynch MP, et al. An interdisciplinary approach to manage cancer cachexia. *Clin J Oncol Nurs.* 2010;14(1):72–80.

96. Kroenke CH, Chen WY, Rosner B, Holmes MD. Weight, weight gain, and survival after breast cancer diagnosis. *J Clin Oncol.* 2005;23(7):1370–1378.

97. Saylor PJ, Smith MR. Adverse effects of androgen deprivation therapy: defining the problem and promoting health among men with prostate cancer. *J Natl Compr Canc Netw.* 2010;8(2):211–223.

Index

Note. *t* refers to a table.